AIDS, CANCER AND THE MEDICAL ESTABLISHMENT

AIDS, CANCER AND THE MEDICAL ESTABLISHMENT

RAYMOND KEITH BROWN, M.D.

ROBERT SPELLER
Publishers
New York, New York 10010

Library of Congress Card
Catalog Number 85-090528
ISBN 0-8315-0196-0

First Edition

Printed in the United States of America
Enquire Printing and Publishing Co., Inc.

This book is dedicated to

DAVID MACDONALD STEWART
1920-1984

Patriot   Philanthropist   Humanitarian

CONTENTS

ACKNOWLEDGEMENTS

I have not included a bibliography for this book, but I have been especially influenced by Hans Selye's THE STRESS OF LIFE and his IN VIVO, Max Gerson's A CANCER THERAPY, and Allan Cantwell's AIDS, THE MYSTERY & THE SOLUTION. Respectively, the McGraw-Hill Book Company, the Liveright Publishing Company, Charlotte Gerson, and Allan Cantwell have given me permission to quote from these invaluable sources. Although I have not quoted from June Goodfield's AN IMAGINED WORLD, (Harper & Row) it classically illustrates the process of scientific discovery, particularly that dealing with iron metabolism and the immune system. I have been also a long time admirer of the brilliant perceptions and researches of Virginia Livingston-Wheeler, so well presented in her 1972 book CANCER, A NEW BREAKTHROUGH. I am especially grateful to Dr. Barrie Cassileth for allowing me to quote liberally from her article on alternative cancer therapies.

I would like to thank Mrs. René Dubos for permission to quote Dr. Dubos, Simon & Schuster for the quotation from Viktor E. Frankl's THE UNHEARD CRY FOR MEANING and W.B. Saunders Company for the quotations from Dr. Colin MacLeod and Sir F. Macfarlane Burnet. I also wish to thank the following for permission to use their letters as appendices to specific chapters: Dr. Alan S. Rabson, Dr. Marlys Witte, Dr. Boguslow Lipinski, Perry A. Chapdelaine, Sr., Edgar Benditzky, and the Guy Owen's family for Dr. Owens letter on pleomorphic organisms. I would also like to thank the Benjamin/Cummings Company for the use of the title page from Domingue's CELL WALL DEFICIENT BACTERIA. (Addison-Wesley Publishing Company).

To thank and acknowledge the friends and acquaintances who have contributed to the evolution of this book goes far beyond the confines of the book itself. There are so many who have contributed to my accumulation of odd bits of knowledge from my practice and other assorted medical activities.

My children, David, Keith and Shannon, with forbearance and love have encouraged me in my rather eclectic path; this I could not have followed were it not for the unfailing friendship and interest of the late David Stewart of Canada.

I am indebted to Drs. Bill Regelson and Lloyd Old, whose unique perceptions and qualities of mind have meant much to me at specific times. Helen Coley Nauts of the Cancer Research Institute has long been a source of inspiration and help. I am grateful to Ed Schlesinger whose interest and legal expertise were comforting to a stranger in New York.

I have been especially appreciative of the unfailing interest and friendship of Ethel Pratt, Lucia Davidova, Elizabeth Harlan Derby, Buell Mullen, Don Papon, Hans Maeder, Mary Ubakivi, Tina Creelman, and the Clinton Curtis and Fred Fayette families.

For specific encouragement and help in the circumstances of this book, I am indebted to Dorothea Seeber of the Independent Citizens Research Foundation, Tom May, Tansey Horn, Bob Anthoine, and those on the 1984 AIDS symposium, from which this book originated. The stars of this show were: Audrey Fjelda, Allan Cantwell, Helen Nauts, Barry Flint, Michael Smith, and especially Lida Mattman, probably the most knowledgable and fascinating current authority on pleomorphic organisms.

I am especially appreciative for the long standing friendship and professional advice of Ruth Aley. I am also indebted to Ken Heuer for his encouragement and valuable suggestions. My especial gratitude goes to Antonio, who designed the book cover, to Polly Horn who helped me in my last minute revisions and to Katherine Hoch for copy editing my manuscript.

Last, but far from least, I owe so much to my patients, especially those with AIDS or cancer. They have taught me and contributed so much, and most of them have also been my friends. With genuine affection, I salute them.   RKB

1

WHAT THIS BOOK IS ABOUT

This book began in September 1984 when I helped organize a small symposium for physicians and workers interested in the broad picture of AIDS. It has evolved into three interwoven themes.

(1) I have presented some of the approaches outside of orthodoxy which may be beneficial in the prevention and control of AIDS. Although the tragedy of AIDS is beyond a simple cause or solution, its outlook is not invariably as dismal as official statistics indicate. I discuss the evidence that the AIDS virus is primarily an additional and catalytic co-factor, precipitating clinical disease only in those whose body defenses are already compromised or defective. I present the reasons that AIDS should be officially recognized as three separate but related disease states rather than the two generally accepted ones.

(2) My second theme presents larger aspects of medicine that are officially unrecognized and controversial. These generally relate to AIDS. Foremost among them are pleomorphic (cell wall deficient) organisms that appear to bridge the gap between bacteria and viruses. The existence in Canada of a microscope capable of working with living cells in magnifications overlapping those of electron microscopy demonstrate the existence of these organisms unequivocally. I am privileged to present previously

unpublished and unavailable photographs made with this microscope of organisms taken from patients with cancer and AIDS.

(3) AIDS, as a distillation of what cancer has long symbolized, leads to my third theme, the tug of war between the Medical Establishment and those who use alternative health and medical approaches to disease. The tensions and conflicts between their philosophies have been issues periodically raised in Washington. I present the inflexibilities of our medical institutions as they are demonstrated by The National Institutes of Health (NIH) and the Food and Drug Administration (FDA). The results of the NIH's narrow specialization in research, and in funding research programs in other institutions, have been disappointing when applied to AIDS. The FDA'S "proof of efficacy" requirements for all health and medical products are the reason that many therapies pertinent to AIDS are unavailable to physicians in the United States.

One of my concerns is to present for the intelligent and curious reader a perspective to the medical iceberg whose visible tip is AIDS. I have placed in the Appendix various items that, although not essential to the themes I have presented, provide in more detail what I have touched on in the book.

2

APOLOGIA

As a pragmatic country doctor for two decades I used non-specific bacterial vaccines for a wide area of disease. There were honorable academic antecedents for their usage, going back to the turn of the century when infection was considered the primary cause of disease, and resistance to infection the sole purpose of the immune system. The mid-century introduction of antibiotics diverted academic interest from the field so the 1970s abolition of bacterial vaccines by the FDA affected only a minority of physicians and their patients. I found beneficial results in a wide spectrum of chronic conditions, ranging from croup, asthma, multiple sclerosis, psoriasis and many forms of arthritis. I was encouraged in my interests by numerous individual physicians throughout the country, whom I found through the pharmaceutical representatives of the companies which produced the vaccines. Foremost among these was the late Dr. K.A. Baird, allergist of St. John, New Brunswick, Canada. This grand old man had devoted his professional life to a futile attempt at gaining official recognition of this type of therapy. His classic "The Human Body and Bacteria" was serially published in the May to November 1966 issues of THE REVIEW OF ALLERGY.

I had developed an awareness of the clinical potentials of vitamin therapy in medical school when I found that the neuritis, eye inflammation, nasal pimples and cracked lip corners I suffered almost every summer under heat and physical stress could be treated and prevented by Vitamin B complex. In practice I subsequently found that many of the clinical claims advanced for Vitamins C and E were justified when I tried them on my patients. Discovering that many baffling and bizarre neuropsychiatric conditions were amenable to dietary restrictions and control of environmental allergens, I found myself in the camp of health oriented physicians, using many pragmatic therapies for which there was little official recognition. I also became aware of the total lack of interest in these therapies by physicians in clinical specialties and academic research.

After leaving general practice, I discovered the academic institutions, with which I became affiliated, had a similar unconcern for alternative therapies. In cancer, I found an often concealed but generally present hostility to any therapeutic approaches outside the control and approval of the Medical Establishment. As I had experience with bacterial vaccines, one of my duties was to investigate these cancer alternatives. Consequently I was privileged to develop a rather comprehensive acquaintance with the field and its usually colorful, sometimes brilliant and often difficult researchers and clinicians. My experiences were augmented by my subsequent association with a large philanthropic foundation that had wide interests in health, nutrition and medical research.

In 1982 I completed a book extensively reviewing alternatives in health and medicine but no editor matched my enthusiasm for it. I therefore took the advice of an interested publisher that I should obtain publicity for my work by clinically demonstrating the value of its contents. As AIDS was emerging to wide attention at the time, I put my book on the shelf and became interested in AIDS.

I found that although AIDS is a horror to those who are its victims, it is the ultimate challenge to those interested in the medical scene. AIDS involves politics, sociology, psychology, public health and sex. It extends across general medicine, microbiology and immunology and shares many aspects of degenerative disease (cancer, arthritis, cardiovascular conditions and collagen disease).

I have treated a number of patients, learned from them, and some of them I have helped. Interviewing and following the clinical courses of others, I have been especially interested in comparing patients who have chosen health alternatives with those treated conventionally. I have been especially interested in the psycho-social aspects of the immune system, particularly applied to the progression of clinical AIDS.

My original book remains on the shelf and AIDS, CANCER AND THE MEDICAL ESTABLISHMENT, incorporating many of its observations and some of its contents, has emerged in its place.

I consider this book in the tradition of the pamphleteers whose controversial tracts concerned contemporary issues; often these were effective in directing attention of the public and the actions of its leaders to areas and issues previously unnoted and ignored.

3

THE DIVISIONS OF MEDICINE

There are few individuals who do not have opinions and strong feelings pertaining to medical care within the United States. The AIDS crisis has focused attention on the medical profession, the services it provides, and the general inadequacies of the Medical Establishment in meeting the challenges of today.

Medicine is usually regarded as a monolithic profession and few are aware of its distinct divisions. These can be represented as overlapping circles, much like the Ballantine Ale trademark or the Olympics logos, with the separate spheres often competing for the shared center. As pertinent to the problems and treatment of AIDS as to all major diseases are the three major aspects of today's medicine:

The first is modern SCIENTIFIC MEDICINE, the legally established standard by which all healing arts and practices are judged and upon which the institutions of the Medical Establishment are based. Centered in hospitals and laboratories, its clinical practices rely heavily on chemical pharmacology and technology. Scientific medicine is measurable, authoritarian and expensive; its treatments for ill health and chronic disease have not matched its successes with acute and surgical conditions. Its failure to provide adequate, humane and reasonably priced

6

primary care to the general public has increasingly generated dissatisfaction and concern among the public and has led to much legislative activity by the government.

HEALTH ORIENTED MEDICINE, the second aspect, aligns with the more physiologic and patient-centered traditions of Hippocrates and of Osler (probably the most eminent medical educator and clinician of this century). Oriented to both internal and external environmental conditions, it emphasizes the innate healing ability of the body. It attempts to strengthen body defenses with a pharmacology largely composed of the natural components of the body. These include enzymes, hormones, minerals, vitamins and other nutrients. Health Oriented Medicine places the responsibility for good health more on the individual than on the medical profession. Its practices are increasingly supported by an interested public that has previously had few alternatives to the care provided by the Medical Establishment. Representing a secularizing trend in medicine, it aligns with much that is advocated and disseminated by the Health Movement. Much of the substance of Health Oriented Medicine is included in the term "preventive medicine". Many of its practices and the physicians who use them are strongly contested by the Medical Establishment that perceives them as a threat to the established order of its institutions.

The third aspect, HOLISTIC MEDICINE, goes beyond the physical boundaries of Scientific or of Health Oriented Medicine. Relating to the ancient inseparabilities of mind, spirit and body, its energy alignments are primarily derived from Oriental concepts. Acupuncture, biofeedback, homeopathy, psychic healing, Yoga, meditation, and the application of mental and spiritual attitudes and exercises to the healing process are increasingly being recognized by the public. They are more widely used by health practitioners (who are not necessarily medical doctors) than by the medical profession.

These three aspects of medicine and health, while competitive, are neither exclusive nor incompatible. All three together are essential for realizing the potentials of each. It is by combinations of these approaches that, unnoted by either the medical Establishment or the general public, control, improvement, and occasionally remission of AIDS has been achieved in scattered patients. These cases are not included in statistics nor given official recognition; they seldom conform with medical practices sanctioned by the Food and Drug Administration and other medical authorities.

4

AN INTRODUCTION TO AIDS

AIDS (Acquired Immune Deficiency Syndrome) is characterized by a breakdown of the immune system so that infections, tumors, and malignancies to which the body is normally resistant can emerge. It is an infectious but not highly communicable disease with an incubation period that has been estimated from three months to five years. It is primarily transmitted sexually, congenitally, by blood products, and by the use of shared unsterilized hypodermic needles. Officially it is diagnosed only by the presence of Kaposi's sarcoma (a skin tumor of variable malignancy) or by Opportunistic Infection (a wide variety of infections to which humans are usually resistant). Four years of intense medical scrutiny has failed to show any evidence that AIDS is transmitted by food, insects or casual contact between individuals.

The first official case of AIDS was noted in the United States in 1979 but it is now reported from over 71 different countries. There have been more than 15,000 reported cases in the United States, and approximately half of them have died. There has been wide media coverage of its high mortality rate, distressing clinical course and generally poor response to treatment. These have created public consternation and fears like those from leprosy, the plague, and Syphilis in other times. There has been little scientific evidence to justify this fear for those outside the

9

major risk groups; the inhumanity that has been so evident, particularly toward pediatric victims, has been more appropriate to the herd instincts of the barnyard than to a supposedly rational and civilized nation.

AIDS first surfaced to public attention in 1981 within the homosexual communities of New York and San Francisco; it has been subsequently identified in intravenous drug users, in hemophiliacs and other recipients of blood or blood products, in infants and children from homes in which there is an AIDS patient and in the sexual partners of those with AIDS or at risk of AIDS. Aids is also found in scattered patients who do not fit the foregoing risk categories. The specter of a widening involvement outside these groups, as in Central Africa (where more than fifty percent of the cases reported are in women) has caused increasing concern and apprehension to many, but events have not justified the fear.

A Special Report on the AIDS Epidemic published in the 29 Feb. 1985 issue of the New England Journal of Medicine presented an awesome review of the current status of AIDS in the United States. It estimated that at least 400,000 persons are now infected with the HTLVIII-LAV virus (which is now generally regarded as the cause of AIDS) and thus at risk of developing the disease. This estimate is now regarded as being too conservative and a million infected persons is considered more accurate. The report cited the Center for Disease Control estimate that there will be a total of 40,000 AIDS cases by the end of 1988. It noted that there are apparently healthy carriers from whom the virus can be cultured although they have no laboratory or physical evidence of disease. The review comments that the complete clinical spectrum of AIDS associated disease is unknown. Also unknown is the percentage of this group which will have malignancies (particularly lymphomas) which are often associated with AIDS. Noting the magnitude of stress that AIDS imposes on current health care systems, the report estimates that the total cost of AIDS to society will be in the billions each year.

There are parallels between today's emergence of AIDS and the appearance of Syphilis in 15th century Europe. Despite many theories (the most widely held is that Syphilis was brought from the New World by the crew of Columbus), there is persuasive evidence that it began in Africa as an infection of certain animal species which by some genetic transformation crossed into the human vector and sexually surged throughout the world. AIDS has also emerged out of Africa, with disability and terror in its wake.

It is believed that the AIDS virus possibly reached the United States from Haiti. In the early '70s Haiti supplied a large number of workers to Zaire, in the center of Africa, where AIDS has subsequently been widely found. It is generally thought that the returning workers brought the virus home with them. Here a severely malnourished population, immunosuppressed from their loads of viral, parasitic and tubercular infections, provide a background on which the AIDS virus can produce disease.

It has been theorized that the AIDS virus was introduced into the gay community of the United States by vacationers to Haiti who were infected there by Haitian men engaged in part-time prostitution. In view of their cultural and religious background, many of these latter were unable to admit their homosexual participation when they subsequently developed AIDS. It is now felt that many Haitian men with AIDS probably belong within the homosexual risk group. That the incidence of AIDS antibody titer has not increased within the Haitian population of the United States comparable to the increased incidence among homosexuals, hemophiliacs and intravenous drug users, renders more convincing the propriety of removing Haitians from the "at risk of AIDS" category.

That AIDS has been centered predominantly among homosexuals and intravenous drug users has emotionally charged the issue so that politicians have approached it gingerly. Responding to the increasing political strength of far-right religious groups in Washington (who view it as a moral rather than a health issue), the White House has generally ignored it; there have been no conferences sponsored by any governmental agency for those providing health and medical care for AIDS patients.

The identification of the agent causing AIDS has been the challenge of the decade. The medical news event of 1984 was the isolation of an organism by Dr. Luc Montaigner and his French group at the Institute Pasteur and by Dr. Robert Gallo and his United States group at the National Institute of Health. This virus, which they respectively termed Lymphadenopathy Virus (LAV) and Human T-Cell Leukemia Virus III (HTLVIII), has been demonstrated to be present in almost all AIDS cases. There is general scientific agreement that these retroviruses (a general grouping that contains the enzyme marker reverse transcriptase) are substantially the same although there are reservations concerning the sub-group to which they belong.

Dr. Gallo and his group maintain they are members of the HTLV (Human T-Cell Leukemia Virus) family which they discovered in 1980, while Dr. Montaigner and his group have placed them within the Lente virus family, which has been demonstrated to produce illness in animals but not previously in humans. The determination of the family to which they belong will decide whether Gallo or Montaigner receives the ultimate recognition as discoverer of the AIDS virus.

Among the excitement and congratulations generated by their discoveries, it has been generally overlooked that the HTLVIII-LAV virus (or AIDS VIRUS, as, for convenience, it will be referred to in this book) is only the precipitating agent, the catalyst, in the AIDS process and by itself does not directly cause the disease. There have been few cases of AIDS where there has not been evidence of other or previous infection by viruses, bacteria, fungi or protoza.

5

THE CATEGORIES OF AIDS

Officially, and for the majority of physicians, the term AIDS applies only to patients belonging to a risk group with immunosuppression manifest by Kaposi's sarcoma, Opportunistic Infection or both. Generally and unofficially, AIDS Related Complex has been considered a precursor of AIDS, although it is now recognized valid for only the twenty percent of cases who progress to KS. or Opportunistic infection. A logical action would be to place ARC within the official AIDS category; this would give the following separate but related categories, ranging from threatening to serious to catastrophic:

(1) The first category is AIDS Related Complex (ARC) whose most common characteristic, enlarged lymph nodes (called Lymphadenopathy Syndrome in Europe) is usually but not invariably present. ARC is probably best considered an individualized response of the body to a variety of stimulae that include the AIDS virus.

ARC includes those patients within the population at risk (homosexuals, intravenous drug users and hemophiliacs) who have clinical symptoms for which no specific cause can be found. These can include fever, weight loss, diarrhea, general fatigue and feelings of unwellness, enlarged and tender lymph nodes, headaches and mental changes. Laboratory studies are suggestive

13

but not absolutely diagnostic. They can include low white blood cell counts, especially among the T-lymphocyte population with a reversal of helper/suppressor (T4T/8) ratios, poor to absent 24 hour skin test reactions to standardized antigens, and an elevation of the blood sedimentation rate (a non-specific indication of disturbed body functioning).

Evidence of present or past viral infections with Hepatitis B, Cytomegalic, Epstein-Barr and Herpes viruses are almost always present as are parasites and fungi (most often Candida). No case of AIDS has been found that does not have several or all of these conditions. It appears likely that all ARC patients harbor portions of the AIDS virus within their systems but the degree and duration of its infectivity is not known, nor whether it can ever be completely eliminated from the body. It may possibly be seeded in the tissues throughout the body, like inactive tuberculosis, awaiting conditions favorable to its reactivation.

Retrovirus infections in animals are persistent, often lifelong, and there is little reason to doubt that this also applies to the Aids virus in humans. Almost all blood donors, from whom recipients have acquired infection leading to AIDS, were asymptomatic at the time they donated blood. The AIDS virus has been isolated from them from one month to five years later.

Whether AIDS Related Complex progresses to Kaposi's sarcoma or Opportunistic Infection depends on the defense mechanisms of the body. These are directly influenced by nutritional status, enzyme, hormonal and acid-base balances of the body, by tissue oxidation, genetic factors and the presence and amount of accessory infections. Stress from the latter is added to that of emotional factors.

Failure to include AIDS Related Complex as a form of AIDS is a statistical convenience for the CDC (Center for Disease Control) but a disservice to all concerned with the implications of the AIDS virus. It is comparable to excluding all patients from the diagnosis of Tuberculosis unless they are hemorrhaging from the lungs.

Almost all ARC patients are considered to have had contact with or to harbor the AIDS virus although less than 20 percent of them progress to Kaposi's sarcoma or Opportunistic Infection. It is unlikely that anyone has developed either of these conditions from the AIDS virus alone.

Some patients have developed symptoms resembling acute mononucleosis shortly after exposure to the virus, either from needle stick (rarely) or sexual exposure. They can have fever, sore throat, malaise, gastrointestinal symptoms, muscle aches and generalized involvement of their lymph nodes. This picture often accompanies the development of a positive antibody response to the AIDS virus, and is transient in a healthy person.

General health measures improve body defenses and may help prevent or modify the effects associated with the AIDS virus. The failure to classify ARC as AIDS may justify conventional medical policy of watchful waiting for the emergence of Kaposi's sarcoma or Opportunistic Infection but it also justifies the actions of those patients who investigate and use all available measures to help maintain or restore health to their bodies.

(2) The second category, Kaposi's sarcoma, holds a unique and possibly misleading place in the field of cancer, as well as in AIDS. In the past, classic Kaposi's sarcoma has been considered a generally benign tumor of the skin and sometimes of the intestinal tract, usually found in elderly males of Mediterranean (usually Italian) or Jewish ancestry. It normally runs an indolent course and is satisfactorily treated or contained by irradiation or local excision. In the past decade, Kaposi's sarcoma has been reported to accompany immunosuppressive drug therapy of organ transplants or collagen disease; when the drugs are stopped, the lesions often regress. Kaposi's sarcoma has also been endemic in certain African areas; lately a particularly aggressive inflam-

matory variety is in evidence there, resistant to therapy and closely resembling AIDS-associated Kaposi's in this country.

The lesions of Kaposi's sarcoma are tumors (any overgrowth of tissue) but they seldom conform to the characteristics of malignancy* Although classed as a sarcoma (a malignant lesion derived from connective tissue), Kaposi's sarcoma does not generally fit this picture. It is usually considered to be formed from endothelial cells which line blood vessels and lymphatics; it seldom metastasizes (spreads through the body by the lymphatics or the blood stream), which is the hallmark of most malignancies.

The mechanisms for the formation of Kaposi's sarcoma are still unknown although there is evidence that Cytomegalic and Epstein-Barr viral infections are involved. That classic Kaposi's sarcoma arising from immunosuppressive medication can spontaneously resolve when the medicine is withdrawn supports the evidence that it is not usually malignant. That these patients develop Kaposi's and not Opportunistic Infection also suggests that their basic mechanisms are different. In the laboratory, the mononuclear cells of Kaposi patients behave like cells from normal controls, being capable of producing alpha-Interferon when stimulated by the Herpes virus; those from patients with Opportunistic Infections are unable to do so. It has been suggested that immunosuppression may not be the direct cause of Kaposi's sarcoma but that it permits secondary infection by micro-organisms that aid in producing the lesions.

AIDS-associated Kaposi's sarcoma has been treated as a malignancy with varying and usually temporary success. The primary treatments have been Interferon, Interleukon 2, other immunomodulators, and chemotherapy. Although sometimes successful in shrinking the lesions, these agents usually have undesirable side effects and little effectiveness in reversing im-

---

*Chapter 19

munosuppresion, the major feature of AIDS. The ardor of those advocating chemotherapy has been somewhat dampened by its immunosuppressive side effects which further diminish the already low defenses of the patient.

Medicine needs to distinguish between Kaposi's sarcoma and Opportunistic Infection. Although they frequently co-exist, lumping them together as a single disease is statistically convenient but scientifically and morally indefensible. The three year mortality for Kaposi's sarcoma alone is fifteen percent; telling a patient who has only Kaposi's sarcoma "You have AIDS which has an eighty percent two year mortality rate" is morally indefensible and a distortion of fact. It frequently damages the patient by pushing him into a severe depression or into too enthusiastic treatment programs; either of these can further depress what little immune reserves he might possess. The reason for the increased rate of Kaposi's sarcoma among homosexuals compared to other risk groups has not been determined.

(3) Opportunistic Infection, the third category of AIDS, either with or without Kaposi's sarcoma is the basis for the usually dismal prognosis of those who have AIDS. Multiple infections (viral, protozoal, fungal and bacterial) are the rule with regular and overlapping recurrences despite therapy for the individual infections. In this country, Pneumocystis Carinii pneumonia is the most common Opportunist Infection while in undeveloped countries, mycobacterial infections and fungi are frequent.

With Opportunistic Infection, the function and regeneratory capacity of lymphocytes, the main arm of the immune system, are depressed, or destroyed, as are other aspects of the body defense systems. Metabolic, endocrine and enzyme functions disintegrate throughout the liver, lungs, adrenals, the gastrointestinal tract and the nervous system. Malignancies, particularly lymphomas and squamous cell carcinomas of the skin, are frequent. Lymph node biopsies show a depletion of all structural elements. Defective immunoglobulin can produce autoimmune phenomena by interacting with body tissues to produce kidney disease and low platelet counts (often manifest as thrombocytopenic purpura, a defect of the bleeding mechanism).

The treatment of Opportunistic Infection has primarily been with chemical agents and antibiotics against whatever causative organisms can be demonstrated, and with supportive therapy for whatever conditions demand attention (ie: blood and platelet transfusions, intravenous feedings and replacement of fluids, minerals and vitamins lost by diarrhea or disturbed nutrition). Gamma globulin has been shown to maintain pediatric patients free from recurrent Pneumocystis pneumonia although it does not alleviate the underlying immunosuppression.

The most common opportunistic infections are Pneumocystis Carinii pneumonia, Avian Tuberculosis, Toxoplasmosis and Cryptosporidiosis. Monilial (Candida) infection is widely prevalent as a lesser opportunistic infection; its presence suggests but is not generally diagnostic of AIDS although there are increasing indications that it may play a larger role in AIDS and other degenerative diseases than has been generally recognized.

An association of human Tuberculosis with AIDS has been widely noted. It has been suggested that its presence in the risk segments of the population should be considered "lesser AIDS"; this tentative category would include Herpes Zoster (Shingles), oral Candidiasis (a yeast infection) and idiopathic thrombocytopenia (low platelet count).

THE LANCET, JANUARY 1/8, 1983

Letters to the Editor

GENERALISED KAPOSI'S SARCOMA IS NOT A NEOPLASM

SIR,—Kaposi's sarcoma has lately achieved notoriety through an epidemic of the generalised form among homosexual males in the United States. Some patients presented with diffuse lymphadenopathy and/or opportunistic infections also but the features in common were an acquired immunodeficiency syndrome (AIDS) and reversal of the normal ratio of helper to suppressor T lymphocytes. Intravenous drug abusers, Haitian immigrants, and haemophiliacs are also at risk.[1]

The epidemic of the generalised form of Kaposi's sarcoma among patients with AIDS is regarded by many as an opportunity to gain insight into the pathogenesis, prophylaxis and treatment of neoplasia.[2] That may well be so but the idea that Kaposi's sarcoma, in its disseminated form, is not a neoplasm is seldom considered. Sarcomas are usually derived from mesenchymal cells. They present as a single mass and metastasise via the blood, first to the lung in most cases. The rarer sarcomas that are derived from the endothelium or other vascular cells fit this pattern too.[3] The origin of Kaposi's sarcoma, seems to be endothelium.[4,5] Histopathologically the lesions of Kaposi's sarcoma are consistent with a benign proliferation of the endothelium—indeed in its incipient phases the lesion is not easy to differentiate from granulation tissue or stasis dermatitis. Infiltration of the connective tissue matrix by proliferating cells is seen in benign endothelial tumours and it is a feature of tissue vascularisation. Tumour-like proliferations of endothelium with a microscopic appearance simulating a sarcoma have been described,[6] these lesions behave benignly.

Even proponents of the malignant nature of the Kaposi lesion will accept that the many affected sites seen in the generalised form of the disease represent multicentric involvement rather than metastasis. Our studies (unpublished) on material kindly supplied by Dr H. Falk and Dr T. Spire have revealed that affected lymph nodes in homosexual men presenting with diffuse adenopathy sometimes contain minute, capsular, and sinusoidal Kaposi lesions accompanied by lymphoid hyperplasia. This is not typical of metastatic involvement. Similarly, when the pulmonary parenchyma is involved, the lesion is found in the bronchial septa and probably involves the bronchial vessels—a very different picture from the typical pulmonary nodules seen in metastatic sarcomas, including angiosarcomas.

It is tempting to draw parallels between Kaposi's sarcoma and infectious mononucleosis (IM), a benign multicentric, and polyclonal lymphoproliferative lesion, which in some cases mimics a malignant disease histologically, especially in immunosuppressed patients. Death in a patient with IM or generalised Kaposi's sarcoma is more often due to complications of tissue involvement, such as splenic rupture (in IM) or gastrointestinal bleeding (in Kaposi's), than to involvement and/or functional compromise of vital organs by tumour bulk. The parallel becomes even more tantalising when one considers the evidence linking cytomegalovirus (CMV) infection to Kaposi's sarcoma. Could an endothelium-seeking strain of CMV, or even Epstein-Barr virus itself, induce a proliferative capillary lesion with the histological appearance of Kaposi's sarcoma?

Regarding generalised Kaposi's sarcoma as a multicentric proliferative lesion of the endothelium would not exclude the possibility of malignant transformation. Emergence of lymphoma from IM has been reported.[8] It would not be surprising if malignant lesions in Kaposi's sarcoma patients were to arise most often in an immunodeficient population.

Laboratory of Pathology,
National Cancer Institute,
National Institutes of Health,
Bethesda, Maryland 20205, U S A,
and Institute Pathology,
C H U Vaudois,
Lausanne, Switzerland

Laboratory of Pathology,
N C I, Bethesda

JOSE COSTA

ALAN S. RABSON

1. Centers for Disease Control MMWR 1982; 31: 507–14
2. Groopman JE, Gottlieb MS Kaposi's sarcoma an oncology looking glass Nature 1982; 299: 103–04
3. Rosenberg SA, Suit HD, Baker LH, Rosen G Sarcomas of soft tissue and bone In DeVita VT, Hellman S, Rosenberg SA, eds Principles in practice of oncology Philadelphia J B Lippincott 1982
4. Nadji M, Morales AR, Ziegler-Weissman J, Penneys NS Kaposi's sarcoma Immunohistologic evidence for an endothelial origin Arch Pathol Lab Med 1981; 105: 274–75
5. Steiny W, Stegelder G K, Bodeux F Kaposi's sarcoma Venous capillary hemangioblastoma Arch Dermatol Res 1979; 266: 253–267
6. Rosai J, Akerman LR Intravenous atypical vascular proliferation a cutaneous lesion simulating a malignant blood vessel tumour Arch Dermatol 1974; 109: 714–17
7. DeVita W, Curran J, Henle W, Johnson Is Workshop on Kaposi's sarcoma Meeting report Cancer Treat Rep 1982; 66: 138–90

8. Abo W, Kamada M, Motoya T, et al Evolution of infectious mononucleosis into Epstein-Barr virus carrying monoclonal malignant lymphoma Lancet 1982; i: 1272–75
9. Wallace JI, Coral FS, Rinman IJ, et al T-cell ratios in homosexuals Lancet 1982; i: 908
10. Gottlieb S, Schroff R, Schanker HM, et al Pneumocystis carinii pneumonia and mucosal candidiasis in previously healthy homosexual men evidence of a new acquired cellular immunodeficiency N Engl J Med 1981; 305: 1425–31
11. Masur H, Michelis MA, Greene JB et al An outbreak of community acquired Pneumocystis carinii pneumonia Initial manifestation of cellular immune dysfunction N Engl J Med 1981; 305: 1431–38
12. Friedman Kien AE, Laubenstein L, Rubenstein P, et al Disseminated Kaposi's sarcoma in homosexual men Ann Intern Med 1982 (no 6, part I)
13. Mildvan D, Mathur U, Enlow R, et al Opportunistic infections and immuno deficiency in homosexual men Ann Intern Med 1982 96 (no 6, part I): 700–04
14. Kornfeld H, Vande Stouwe RA, Lange M et al T-lymphocyte subpopulations in homosexual men N Engl J Med 1982; 307: 729–34
15. Siegal FP, Lopez C, Hammer GS Severe acquired immunodeficiency in male homosexuals, manifested by chronic perianal ulcerative herpes simplex lesions N Engl J Med 1981; 305: 1439–44
16. Curran J, CDC study Reported at American Society of Microbiology meeting (Sept 1st 1982; New York City)

6

THE NINETY PERCENT

The life styles and practices of intravenous drug users and many of the homosexual community have been the background for ninety percent of American AIDS patients. They also relate directly or indirectly to the ten percent of cases found in other population groups.

The distinction between those who get AIDS and those who transmit it is still unknown. There is suggestive evidence that patients with AIDS Related Complex (ARC), as well as asymptomatic carriers of the AIDS virus, are the chief vectors for the transmission of the virus. An early British study of homosexual constellations (groups of sexually interacting individuals) suggested that direct sexual contact between AIDS victims is generally low. This accorded with Dr. Gallo's comment that "There are healthy carriers of AIDS" and "people who already have AIDS probably aren't contagious; there's almost no virus left in them. It's the people who are in the early phases that are infective."

The presence of antibodies to the AIDS Virus does not mean that the person has AIDS, will develop AIDS or is necessarily capable of transmitting AIDS, only that the possibility for all three is present. To complicate the picture further, there are an appreciable number of individuals from whom the AIDS Virus can be cultured but who have no antibody levels nor any laboratory or physical evidence of its presence within their bodies. This carrier state is one of the many perplexing aspects of the disease and may relate to a Scandinavian study; this showed gay men with evidence of suppressed immune responses had twenty times the incidence of antibody to the AIDS virus as a similar group with normal immune responses. It has been suggested that immunocompromised individuals should be added to the list of "risk groups for AIDS".

In one San Francisco study, antibody to the AIDS virus was found in 92% of patients with generalized lymphadenopathy, in 78% of those with other signs or symptoms suggestive of AIDS (eg: oral candidiasis) but in 100% of those with AIDS or with hematologic abnormalities.

For homosexual men, the risk of exposure to the AIDS virus is greater than it was in the early 1980s because of the increasing number who now have the organism. For both heterosexuals and homosexuals, the greater the number of sexual partners, the greater the incidence of sexually transmitted disease. Any sexual contact with an individual whose infectious status is unknown should be considered a high risk. All individuals with a positive antibody test for AIDS virus should be considered infectious but a negative antibody titre does not mean freedom from infection; the blood does not convert (become positive) until some time after infection has taken place.

The common factor in all cases of AIDS is an underlying deficit of body defenses. The philosophy set forth by Pasteur's alleged dying remarks "Bernard is right. The germ is nothing; the terrain is all" applies unreservedly to AIDS. In the 9 July 1983 Lancet, Drs. Jay Levy and John Zeigler of the University of California proposed that AIDS is itself an opportunistic infection, causing disease only in individuals with already compromised immunity. Their article predicted that evidence of previous contact with the AIDS agent would be found in healthy individuals with functioning immune systems. This theory had little initial response from other researchers but has been validated by subsequent evidence that while almost all AIDS patients have antibodies to the AIDS Virus so also have an increasing majority of homosexuals, hemophiliacs and intravenous drug users, regardless of their health status.

Congenital AIDS and AIDS transmitted by blood products are purely medical problems; in homosexuals and intravenous drug abusers, health factors connected with their life styles and poor hygienic measures play a prominent role. The promiscuous or careless activities of a minority have dispersed intestinal parasites, Hepatitis and the Herpes family (including Cytomegalovirus and Epstein-Barr infections) throughout the gay community. Those whose body defenses are depressed by these, progress to ARC, KS or Opportunistic Infection when they are also infected with the AIDS virus.

Epidemiologically and statistically, it has been found that homosexuals at greatest risk are those who indulge in frequent and promiscuious passive anal sex. Ano-genital coupling is apparently not only a major means of transmitting the AIDS virus but has a role in the sexually transmitted diseases that are now endemic in the gay community. These include Hepatitis-B, Cytomegalovirus, Herpes, Epstein-Barr virus, repeated episodes of venereal disease and the assorted bacterial and parasitic diseases of the intestines that have come to be known as the "Gay Bowel Syndrome". These, the legacy of the 1970s explosion of unrestrained sexual freedom directly correspond to the increased incidence of sexually transmitted diseases among heterosexuals.

One of the physiologic functions of spermatic fluid is to immunosuppress locally the female genital tract, thus ensuring that the sperm is not rejected as a foreign protein. Studies have demonstrated that the repeated injection of a mouse with mouse spermatic fluid produces a generally immunosuppressed mouse. It has been medically assumed that AIDS is transmitted into the blood stream by traumatic lacerations or abrasions of the rectal mucosa; it is more logical to consider that spermatic fluid, locally suppressing the rectal mucosa, facilitates its own absorption into the circulation. The generalized immunosuppression it produces is poor protection against the pathogenic organisms also released from containment within the bowel. Antibodies which the body can produce against sperm are also specific against helper (T4) lymphocytes (the integral lymphocyte sub-group that is vital to immunologic function). The T-4 lymphocytes noted to be depressed in many healthy homosexuals, is possibly tied to this mechanism.

Unprotected and promiscuious sexual indulgences are major contributors to the wide spectrum of sexually transmitted illnesses that are a background for AIDS. Although not all AIDS patients have been promiscuious, it follows that the greater the number of sexual partners, the greater is the chance of picking up disease organisms. This applies equally to heterosexual men with AIDS; their multiple exposure to prostitutes apparently equals the statistical promiscuity of many homosexuals with AIDS.

The intravenous drug users disregard for health and safety measures through indiscriminate sharing of dirty syringes and needles has been credited with the high incidence of AIDS within the drug culture. There is no simple explanation for the lower incidence of Kaposi's sarcoma in male compared to female intravenous drug users.

There is unnoted evidence that Heroin is probably as responsible for immunosuppression in this group as careless hygenic measures. Morphine derivatives (especially Heroin when injected into the blood stream) parallel the immunosuppression of spermatic fluid and markedly impair the defenses and functions of body tissues, including resistance to infection. There have been increasing reports of patients on dialysis whose kidneys have been destroyed by Heroin. The addict's disregard for health and safety measures has spread disease (including the AIDS Virus) as effectively as the unprotected sex practices of promiscuous homosexuals. Many in both groups, who now share a common disease, have also shared an unawareness of the effects of their life styles on either themselves or on others.

Any approach to the prevention of AIDS in these two groups must be more than medical. Education and coercion is minimally effective in controlling sexual behavior or drug habits. Legal attempts to regulate or prohibit private behavior and practices, however unhealthy or irresponsible (ie: tobacco and alcohol) is seldom successfull and is contrary to what we consider the inalienable rights of the individual. The gravity of the AIDS epidemic has been sufficient for many in these groups to separate themselves from the careless drug and sexual practices of the '70s. Future AIDS patients from these groups will be those who continue the heedless patterns of the past.

It is unlikely that anti-viral vaccines comparable to the Hepatitis B vaccine can be soon produced to protect against the wide viral components of AIDS. It is also unlikely that a vaccine will be developed against the more than two hundred mutant strains of the AIDS virus that have been identified. The major therapeutic advances will probably be with antimicrobial agents, directed againsts the AIDS virus as well as the associated infections of AIDS.

It appears that the AIDS problem will be only slightly diminished by medical recognition that the AIDS virus precipitates AIDS but is not its sole cause. That either antiviral agents or a vaccine can be developed to protect careless homosexuals and drug users without a change in their motivations and life styles is unlikely. Such a scientific advance would be like the development of a pill allowing one to smoke without risk of lung cancer, heart trouble or emphysema.

7

THE TEN PERCENT

The susceptibility of hemophiliacs to Opportunistic Infection (but not Kaposi's sarcoma) when they have had prolonged treatment with blood products, is largely unexplained. It has been suggested that blood contains an immunosuppressive substance similar to that found in spermatic fluid. A relationship between the clotting mechanism of blood and the immune system is suggested by the high incidence of T4T8 lymphocyte ratio reversals (indicating immunosuppression) found in hemophiliacs using blood products. This is independent of the presence of the AIDS Virus. The currently high incidence of AIDS virus antibodies among hemophiliacs directly relates to the amount of blood products (Factor VIII) they have received. A British study, commenting on the low incidence of AIDS (only 1:1000) among those who demonstrate AIDS virus antibodies points out the superiority of closely monitored Public Health Service blood over that from commercial sources.

The resistance of hemophiliacs is lowered by the unwanted side effects of blood and blood products and the viral pathogens they can introduce. Immunosuppression, possibly associated with blood Factor VIII can also relate to increased iron stores of the body from a breakdown of donated blood cells. There is evidence that free iron adversely affects the function of the immune system and fosters the growth of many organisms and cancer cells.*

It is a reasonable assumption that in Hemophilia: (1) Blood factors, like rectally deposited spermatic fluid and intravenous Heroin, are capable of immunosuppression, regardless of the presence of the AIDS Virus or its antibodies. (2) Immunosuppression from repeated infusions of pooled blood products can increase the hemophiliac's risk of Opportunistic Infection when he eventually comes in contact with the AIDS Virus. (3) The determining factor for the evolution of Opportunistic Infection in such cases is probably the presence of other microbes already present or transmitted through blood products. (4) Kaposi's sarcoma has seldom been reported in hemophiliacs; this suggests a differentiation between Kaposi's sarcoma and Opportunistic Infection. (5 That AIDS Related Complex is not reportable or officially classified as AIDS deprives those in this group and their physicians from consideration of the adjunctive therapies that others find of benefit.

The AIDS-like spectrum of disease in transfused infants, in those born to mothers at risk of AIDS and in those with close familial contact with an AIDS patient, are a deeply distressing but numerically small aspect of the total AIDS picture. Pediatric AIDS relates more to AIDS Related Complex (ARC) and to Opportunistic Infection than to Kaposi's sarcoma which has seldom been reported pediatrically. Due to the prolonged incubation period for AIDS it is now considered that "close familial contact" is probably congenital transmission of the causative agent(s). No family members, household contacts or anyone taking care of pediatric AIDS patients have ever developed evidence of the disease.

The common denominator uniting pediatric categories of AIDS is the developmental immaturity of the newborn and of

---

*page 134

early childhood. This relates to (1) the increased incidence of cancers & leukemia in early childhood. (2) the increased incidence of capillary hemangiomas (blood vessel tumors of the skin which usually diminish spontaneously after the first year of life). (3) the susceptibility of infants to croup and crib death.

The underdeveloped immune systems of infants is probably equivalent to surgery-associated immunosuppression. Both conditions allow the growth of poorly recognized microbes that can later produce much illness. The microbes, usually viral and most often of the Herpes family can contribute their own immunosuppressions concurrently with that of the AIDS Virus. The large number of bacterial infections in these children, as well as Pneumocystis Carinii (the most frequent pediatric opportunist) indicate their B-lymphocyte mediated humoral immunity is also defective.

The development of AIDS following blood transfusions in patients who are not from risk groups can usually be ascribed to the immunosuppression from certain anaesthetic agents and the stress of prolonged surgery. These have been implicated in the high incidence of viral conditions (particularly cytomegalic infections) which can follow prolonged surgery (primarily organ transplants and cardiac surgery).

It appears that women whose sexual partners have transmitted the AIDS organisms to them are comparable to healthy homosexual males, who, harboring the virus, can transmit it and induce AIDS, but only in those whose defenses are inadequate. Women's resistance to clinical AIDS, although they can transmit it to their infants has not been precisely determined. There is the well publicized case of a California prostitute whose four babies (each by a different father) developed AIDS even though she was never diagnosed as having the disease.

There is an increasing incidence of AIDS being reported in prostitutes, with many showing laboratory and physical evidence of AIDS Related Complex. A study of the wives of drug addicts with AIDS has showed similar evidence in many cases. The general resistance of women to AIDS is probably more hormonal than genetic. Estrogen, a stimulant of the reticuloendothelial system of defense, is decreased after the menopause, so women lose their superiority over men in resistance to infectious and degenerative disease.

Serologic determination of AIDS antibody titres should probably be a part of all prenatal check ups. Preventively, there should be meticulous prenatal care for all women who are associated with risk groups, and optimal nutritional care provided for all with underlying health or medical defects. Focusing an equivalent regime on infants born of these women might help prevent or ameliorate illness in some of them. Such preventive measures carry the issue into political areas and would conflict with current cutbacks and elimination of much health and prenatal care for the poor.

An Australian study in the 14 September 1985 Lancet reported that four out of eight women, artificially inseminated from an asymptomatic carrier, developed antibodies to AIDS. Only one had any symptoms and that was a generalized enlargement of her lymph nodes. Three of the women subsequently became pregnant and their babies are, so far, healthy, with no evidence of AIDS antibodies at one years of age. This suggests that healthy women, showing evidence of contact with the AIDS virus, do not necessarily have infected infants.

This report also indicates that the virus can be transmitted by semen implanted in the vagina without trauma or other body contact. There was no history in these women of the acute mononucleosis-like syndrome which has been reported to accompany the development of the AIDS antibody. None of the husbands of these women (presumably also healthy) have developed antibody titers to AIDS in three years. All three children are well even though their mothers definitely had the virus many months before they were conceived. This report suggests that in healthy women, with presumably good body defenses, even the presence of the AIDS virus does not inevitably lead to tragedy. This does not negate the general feeling that women who carry the AIDS virus should not become pregnant.

8

THE PROBLEM OF BLOOD

For the general public, the acquiring of AIDS from blood and blood products is probably the most publicized and disturbing aspect of AIDS, but this fear is out of proportion to the actual incidence of such infection. The risk of developing AIDS is appproximately one in a million transfusions while the risk of death from a transfusion reaction is one in six hundred thousand. Infants receiving blood, due to their underdeveloped immune systems, have five times the chance of developing AIDS as adults.

The currently rigid evaluation of all blood and blood products, and the discarding of all that shows evidence of the AIDS virus or antibodies to it, will eliminate the problem to a major degree. This conflicts with the needs of the blood bank system for adequate blood supplies and also distresses the gay community. The latter perceive that the presence of the AIDS antibodies, besides being a marker for past or current AIDS virus infection might be used as a marker for homosexuality. As an invasion of privacy for blood donors, there could be repercussions in insurance, employment and other avenues of discrimination.

One solution is that all blood should be identified by a code number assigned and given the donor at the time the blood is drawn; the code number would be unrelatable to donor registration with the laboratory. All donors for the day would receive a form letter enclosing the code numbers of rejected bloods; details of rejection would be given only to the donor or his physician upon receipt of the original blood number slip given at donation time.

A positive medical aspect of AIDS will be an increased focus on blood and blood products with an evaluation of their overuse and misuse. Their ready availability and often dramatic immediate results have dimmed an awareness that their often long range ill effects, like the widespread and indiscriminate use of antibiotics, can be ill health and disease. Much blood has previously come from professional donors, often from the lower levels of society and of undetermined health, unscreened except for Syphilis. Current attention to the quality of blood supplies by screening for the AIDS virus and Hepatitis B will, undoubtedly, be directed to other previously ignored microbial components of blood. Limiting blood and blood products only to cases of severe need, and permitting the use of individual blood donors (especially in pediatrics) will curtail the scope and organization of the national blood bank system, but in the long run will benefit the patients.

The immunosuppressive effect of blood and blood products is recognized as beneficial against organ transplant rejection, even as it allows the growth or reactivation of viral infections (especially Cytomegalovirus) within the patient. Still unknown is the reason for the elevated recurrence rate of colon cancer when blood has been given at operation, or the shortened life span of cancer patients who have received blood.

That these conditions may relate to pleomorphic organisms*, present but undetected in the transfused blood, is a still unexplored aspect of medicine.

---

*Chapter 19

9

THE AFRICAN CONNECTION

Africa (where the AIDS virus is believed to have originated) illustrates the Malthusian doctrine that populations tend to increase faster than the means of subsistance, resulting in an inadequate supply of food and necessary goods unless war, famine or disease reduce the number of people in a given area. The AIDS virus, spread largely through the urges and surges of sexuality, is apparently the spark that ignites material prepared by endemic disease, unhealthy life styles and malnutrition.

The nations of central Africa are experiencing an horrendous epidemic of AID. Dependant on tourism as a major source of income, these impoverished countries, with the exception of Rwanda, have downplayed the news, discouraged scientific observers and censored all reports of conditions there. (This closely resembles the situation in which Ethiopia, for political reasons, failed to acknowledge the seriousness of its internal conditions until catastrophic famine enveloped the country.)

The remarks of a major African government official sums up the official attitude: "We prefer to talk about malaria, diarrhea, parasitic diseases and malnutrition, which are our major public health problems". However, these problems pertain directly to AIDS. The immune system is especially sensitive to protein deprivation, which is widely prevalent in Africa and Haiti. Malnutrition, added to Malaria, parasites, and wide microbial infections (largely viral and mycobacterial), provides the conditions on which the AIDS virus flourishes.

African AIDS, affecting the middle and upper income brackets, has produced severe dislocations of the most competent and highly trained people of the involved areas. Community, business and political leaders are affected so that personal tragedies are overshadowed by the effects on the vitality and functioning of business and government.

Dr. William Hasseltine of Harvard Medical School, probably the major authority on African AIDS, has pointed out the deterioration of African health from the crumbling of colonial health structures, extensive population dislocations, and widespread environmental and ecologic disintegration. He estimates that at least ten million people (one tenth of the population) of central Africa are infected with the AIDS virus. This means they carry the AIDS organism in their bodies but it does not mean that they have clinical disease.

Many people fear that the African AIDS epidemic is the harbinger of what is in store for Western nations but this is probably (and hopefully) not justified. It is generally acknowledged that the AIDS virus participates in producing what is essentially the same disease, regardless of geographic location. It is the epidemiology that makes the difference. In African areas where AIDS is prevalent, homosexuality does not appear to be common; there, AIDS is primarily transmitted heterosexually, being almost equally prevalent in men and women.

Rwanda, an exception to the other African countries, has been the source of much information regarding African AIDS. There, a majority of cases are found in the urban areas, and among middle and upper income brackets. Forty percent of cases are among women and twenty two percent among children; this contrasts with the children's rate in the United States of 1.4%. This difference in rates is undoubtedly influenced by the large number of sexually active women there who carry the AIDS virus, and thus transmit it to their infants.

Corresponding to Western patterns of homosexually transmitted AIDS, the risk of heterosexually transmitted AIDS appears to increase with the number of sexual partners, particularly prostitutes. In one study, 80% of the prostitutes had antibody to the AIDS virus, while another study showed only 54%, although 75% of these women showed physical evidence of disease. Another study reported that 43% of women with AIDS were found to be prostitutes. Their high rate of antibodies to the AIDS virus and the many clinical signs and symptoms of AIDS found in African prostitutes, suggest that the latter should be included in the groups at risk for AIDS.

Although sexual promiscuity appears a prominent feature in most of the adult AIDS cases, many of the customs and practices of Africa are not easily investigated or adequately evaluated, especially in rural areas. There, the native practitioners, in response to a general belief in the superiority and efficacy of intravenously administered drugs, use no sterile precautions and the same needle for all. This distribution of multiple infections freely and indiscriminatingly through the population aligns on a wider scale to the habits of the intravenous drug culture in the United States. It has also been noted that, as a social greeting, with no sexual connotation, "tonguing" is widespread as an affectionate greeting among women. This friendly but indiscriminate mixing of saliva can also spread other forms of infection. Both of these practices, as well as the extent of Chlamydial infection (which has an affinity for the lymphatics) might relate to the wide incidence of AIDS among African women. A high incidence of parasitic infection is common within areas affected by AIDS; while immunosuppressed individuals have been noted to be prone to parasitic disease, only recently has the immunosuppressive capacity of almost all parasites been accepted.

The 7 September 1985 issue of The Lancet reports the puzzling association of elevated antibodies against Plasmodium Falciparum (Malaria) and positive AIDS virus antibodies in healthy African natives who show no sign of immunosuppression. No adequate explanation for this seeming paradox has been presented. It is possible that chronic, intermittent and low grade malarial infection in otherwise healthy individuals (like chronic low grade bacterial infection) may stimulate antibodies to prevent the progression of an AIDS virus infection to clinical AIDS. In Uganda, where AIDS has not been reported, 50 out of 75 blood samples drawn for another study in 1972-73 from healthy children, have now been found to have antibody to the AIDS virus.

Heterosexual AIDS in Africa conforms to the 18 Oct. 85 issue of the Journal of the American Medical Association in which Dr. Robert Redfield of Walter Reed Army Hospital reported on the prevalence of HTLVIII Disease treated there. (Significantly, Dr. Redfield included AIDS Related Complex as a part of the AIDS spectrum of disease.) He noted that 15 of their 41 cases were heterosexually transmitted. Six of these patients (women) had contact with men who were at risk of AIDS but the remaining nine (men) had multiple (over 50) heterosexual partners or contacts with prostitutes. Their type of sexual activity did not seem to have any significance for the development of disease; none of them had Kaposi's sarcoma or evidence of active cytomegalic disease. Their sexual promiscuity aligned with those having AIDS in Africa and in the homosexual community.

The highest incidence of AIDS in the United States is found in Belle Glades, Florida, where conditions closely resemble those of Africa where AIDS is prevalent. The population of the migrant and agricultural worker camps are poverty stricken, and often loaded with Tuberculosis, venereal disease, parasites and viruses. The horrors of AIDS are merely additive to the quality of life and of environment found here at this level of society. The distinguishing element of Belle Glade AIDS is that no Kaposi's sarcoma has been reported. Many of the AIDS patients are young unmarried males but neither homosexuality nor intravenous drug use appears to be a feature of their life. So far, there has been no report concerning the health and the AIDS virus status of the prostitutes whom these men patronize.

It may be that Malthusian concepts of the natural remedies for overpopulation are as pertinent to our own urban and rural wastelands as to Africa. The quality of life, the malnutrition and the hopelessness of many who live in these areas might equally relate to their gamut of infections from which AIDS emerges.

10

THE
RETICULOENDOTHELIAL
SYSTEM

The Reticuloendothelial System (RES) is the major and least understood defense system of the body, with its cells dispersed throughout all tissues and organs. The RES encompasses the immune system, but the latter, as the most intellectually challenging and popular object of medical research today, has totally overshadowed the broad dimensions of the RES. It is within the RES and not just the immune system that the devastations of AIDS occur. A classic review of the RES was published by Saba in the Dec 1970 Archives of Internal Medicine.

In the 1880s, Metchnikoff outlined the RES as composed of single cells (including many of the white cells that circulate within blood and lymph vessels) that line the lymph channels of the liver, lung, spleen and bone marrow. They are present within these organs also as fixed connective tissue cells, as well as in skin, adrenals, thyroid, thymus, pituitary and the central nervous system. They maintain the chemical, hormonal and enzymatic balances of the body as well as the adaptive mechanisms described by Selye*, by which the body responds and adjusts to all varieties of stress.

The RES orchestrates and maintains metabolism. This, the

---

*Chapter 18.

sum of the processes by which protoplasm, the living substance of all cells, is produced, maintained and destroyed, produces energy for the cell. The RES also repairs and heals body tissues and immunologically protects against harmful agents from the environment.

The major functions of the RES may be summarized as: Clearing the blood of foreign matter, devitalized tissues and aged red blood cells.

Processing antigens (those substances which stimulate antibody formation) for immunologic ativity.

Metabolizing carbohydrates, fats, proteins and steroids.

Detoxifying drugs and chemicals.

Preventing intravascular clotting.

Inactivating bacterial and chemical toxins.

Activating enzymes.

Synthesizing hemoglobin.

Repairing and healing body tissues.

Among the conditions associated with altered RES function are: shock (from overwhelming infection, hemorrhage or trauma), infection (bacterial, viral, fungal or protozoal), cancer, autoimmune disease, radiation injury, immunologic depression, arteriosclerosis, collagen disease and anemia.

The integrity of the RES depends on a balance between suppression and stimulation. Classic therapy has always emphasized the naturopathic benefits of sunlight, fresh air, pure food and water, cleanliness and tranquillity; the most solid advances in medical therapy have also been those which biologically augment the normal functions of the body. These include vaccination, insulin, vitamins, minerals and hormones, all of which relate to reticuloendothelial function. Many substances, affecting the body through the RES, stimulate in small amounts and are toxic or depressive in large doses. Sunlight stimulates but sunburn blisters. Low doses of chemotherapy, radiation, estrogen, alcohol, heparin, cortisone, insulin and histamine are all reticuloendothelial stimulants. These depress in high doses as do almost all aspects of modern life: viral and parasitic infections, chronic lead poisoning, anoxia (lack of oxygen), hypoglycemia (low blood sugar), sulfur dioxide, hydrocarbons, fluorescent lights, microwaves, and stress of all varieties.

The persistent misuse, often including prolonged use, of antibiotics (and especially the penicillins and tetracyclines) has a triple capacity for mischief. They can suppress the RES, encourage the emergence of antibiotic resistant organisms, and by removing the stimulus of infection to the immune system, impair resistance to subsequent infections. Elimination of much chronic bacterial infection by improved hygiene, vaccinations and antibiotics has probably atrophied our reticuloendothelial systems. In the 4 November 1974 Lancet, Dr. J.A. Raeburn of the University of Edinburgh suggested that the widespread use of antibiotics, especially at crucial stages of fetal development, might, in genetically prone women, produce immunodeficient infants. He noted that these conditions were first reported in 1952 after the use of antibiotics had become widespread. He considered it unlikely that such states had been earlier overlooked from lack of medical knowledge or unavailability of diagnostic tests.

The major defenses of the body, mediated primarily through the reticuloendothelial system, are:

(A) Cell mediated immunity, primarily achieved through the T-lymphocytes processed by the thymus gland.

(B) Humoral immunity, mediated by antibodies from plasma cells, which themselves are derived from B-lymphocytes.

(C) Interferon, a general family of non-specific substances produced in response to varying antigenic stimulation (usually viral or bacterial). Their anti-viral and anti-tumor effects have not been as definite as was first thought but there are many still unexplored forms of Interferon with uncharted activities and complexities. Dr. Klemawesch of Duke University has observed that in cancer patients prolonged Interferon administration produces a significant depression of Complement 3, an essential component of the complement system.

(D) The Complement system, activated by antigen-antibody reactions, an exceptionally complex cascade of enzymatic processes which protects the body against foreign substances, microorganisms and cancer. It is probably the most intensely investigated of any body defense systems but it still has few therapeutic applications.

(E) The phagocytic defense system in which granulocytes (white blood cells with many nuclei, also known as polymorphonuclear cells) and phagocytes (other specialized white blood cells derived from lymphocytes and monocytes and often termed macrophages) engulf and dispose of foreign substances. These include microbes and break-down products of the body.

It is from the granulocytes and macrophages primarily that acute phase substances (collectively termed Interleukin I) produce a wide variety of defense mechanisms that include temperature elevations, C-reactive proteins, alterations of sleep, and shifts and sequestrations of trace minerals within the body. Elevation of blood sedimentation rates in infections, malignancies and other body disturbances are related to this class of reactivity.

(F) The properdin system, a naturally occuring antibody closely allied with Complement 3 and found in plasma (the liquid part of blood or lymph) that helps to confer species resistance to microbial agents and even malignancies. Properdin was extensively researched by Pillimer and associates in the '50s and early '60s but then all interest in it evaporated and it was regarded as having been a figment of Pillimer's imagination. It is again scientifically respectable although not fashionable, so there is little work being done in this field. The enigma of why AIDS has been almost impossible to transmit to animals, including monkeys, by the injection of blood or other material from AIDS patients or by the AIDS Virus, might be that the animals do not have the accessory infections and depressed defense mechanisms that are found in AIDS Patients. The presence of Properdin and an adequate complement system in the animals used are also probably factors in their resistance to infection with the AIDS Virus.

There was wide news coverage when research on the reticuloendothelial system was first presented at the 1959 conference of the New York Academy of Science. There was optimism that stimulation of the body's general defenses by specific substances might be a panacea for conditions ranging from infection to cancer and the degenerative processes. This resembles the optimism of researchers today that specific therapy, working at the T-lymphocyte level, might solve the problems of the wide systemic involvements of AIDS.

Any consideration of AIDS and the reticuloendothelial system is inadequate without knowledge of the liver, which is probably involved in every case of AIDS Related Complex or Opportunistic Infection, and frequently in Kaposi's sarcoma.

Sixty percent of the body's reticuloendothelial cells are inseparable from the hepatic cells of the liver; from them the products of their myriad and still poorly charted metabolic and chemical reactions are carried throughout the body by the blood. Their interrelationships are reflected in the disturbed reticuloendothelial functioning, usually immunologic, from any liver injury. Immunologic and metabolic disturbances are the basis for chronic degenerative diseases, especially those of heart, lung, and from cancer; these caused sixty percent of all deaths reported in 1984 as compared to twelve percent of all deaths in 1900.

Liver disease, including hepatitis and cirrhosis, ranks fifth as a cause of death in the United States; it has been estimated that it will rise to third place within the next decade. We can be pretty sure that the increasing amount of industrial pollution, chemical hazards in an expanding industrial economy, and the development of new drugs have been heavy contributors to the upsurge of liver ailments.

The liver is the largest and only self-regenerating organ of the body, renewing itself when any portion has been destroyed or removed. The ancient Greeks incorporated this characteristic of the liver in their myth of Prometheus bound to the rock; his liver, devoured each day by a vulture, regenerated itself each night.

With the heavily polluted environment and destructive life styles of today, even Prometheus would have difficulty in regenerating his liver. Liver disease must be extensive before it produces laboratory abnormalities, so "normal" liver studies do not necessarily mean a healthy liver. As with advanced cancer, almost all livers are damaged and malfunctioning in AIDS, presumably from Hepatitis or Cytomegalovirus infections. The frequent intolerance of AIDS patients to chemotherapeutic agents well tolerated by other patients, is probably due to their underlying liver dysfunction.

11

THE VIRUSES of AIDS

The major viruses associated with AIDS are Hepatitis B and the Herpes family. The latter includes the three well known varieties (Herpes I, Herpes II, and Herpes Zoster, also known as Shingles). It also includes Cytomegalovirus and the Epstein-Barr virus.

Hepatitis B virus (HBV) infection of the liver is a major health consideration for those groups at risk of AIDS. It is spread by blood products and body fluid, paralleling the transmission of the AIDS Virus. Although it is not confined to homosexuals and intravenous drug users, its greatest prevalence in the United States is within these groups. Its rapid spread in the 1970s (it was uncommon in the United States before then) resembled closely the later dissemination of the AIDS virus. It has been estimated that four to six percent of asymptomatic male homosexuals are carriers, capable of transmitting the infections although eighty five percent are estimated to have been infected by the age of forty. The infectivity of Hepatitis B far exceeds the AIDS virus; it is an occupational hazard for dentists and medical workers (especially surgical teams) who may be accidentally exposed to contaminated blood.

It is estimated that in this country there are 150,000 patients each year with asymptomatic and undetected Hepatitis B infections, approximately 50,000 who have symptoms (including jaundice) but are treatable on an ambulatory basis, 10,000 who require hospitalization, and 250 deaths. One percent (30,000) of the three million patients who yearly receive blood transfusions develop the disease although ten percent (300,000) are estimated to develop undetected hepatitis.

The main danger of Hepatitis B is that it can persist as a chronic disease with disability and ultimately death from cirrhosis, polyarteritis (a poorly understood inflammation of the arteries) or liver cancer. The World Health Organization has reported that liver cancer, the leading cause of cancer death in Africa and China, probably relates to Hepatitis B infections which are endemic in those areas. A large part of the problem there is considered to be the congenital transmission of the infection to infants from chronically infected mothers.

Cirrhosis stemming from Hepatitis-B can be independent of, but strongly additive to, the effects of alcohol. There is evidence of Hepatitis-B involvement in pancreatitis and in pancreatic cancer; it has been found outside the liver in blood vessel walls, in bile ducts, spleen, bone marrow and in white blood cells. Carriers of HBV antibodies (evidence of past infection) have an increased incidence of cancer.

Primarily because of apathy and ignorance, the safe and effective anti-HBV vaccine now available has been poorly accepted. (These two factors also contribute to the tendency of medical authorities to ignore the role of damaged livers and the reticuloendothelial dysfunctions in AIDS.) In most AIDS cases, it is impossible to separate the features of the Hepatitis-B virus and those of the Herpes family (especially the Cytomegalovirus and the Epstein-Barr virus) that blend within the liver and throughout the reticuloendothelial system.

Ogden Nash quipped "God, in His wisdom, made the fly— and then forgot to tell us why". Like flies, herpetic viruses are embedded in our environment although no one has demonstrated their ecologic benefit. It is estimated that each year adds one-half to a million fresh cases of Herpes infection to the twenty million Americans estimated to harbor the virus. The best known forms of Herpes are Herpes Zoster, Herpes I and Herpes II.

In children, Herpes Zoster virus produces Chickenpox (Varicella), a violently contagious skin eruption. After the skin has cleared, the virus is sequestered within the nervous system where it usually remains dormant. In later life it may erupt as Shingles, the unusually painful, often persistent and prostrating skin eruptions of an immune system stressed by age, illness and other vicissitudes of life. It has frequently been noted in risk groups as a forerunner of AIDS.

Undramatic, cosmetically annoying and somewhat painful, fever blisters (cold sores) caused by Herpes Simplex I are found mostly around the mouth; they are, after the initial infection, laid down in the nerves supplying the facial areas. They appear thereafter as fresh eruptions during periods of either physical or emotional stress. Herpes I has been generally considered innocuous except when, involving the branches of the trigeminal nerve that supply the surface of the eye, it results in corneal ulceration or scarring. However, Herpes I is increasingly recognized as a cause of viral meningitis and encephalitis.

Herpetic eye infections are one of the dilemmas of medical treatment where diagnosis is of the highest importance. Cortisone and its analogues have been the drug of choice for Zoster but can produce sight-threatening complications when used for Herpes Simplex. Acyclovir is now the drug of choice and the prototype of antiviral drugs; it can modify or abort the immediate lesion but it does not cure the underlying infection.

Before the recognition of Chlamydial infection, genital herpes, caused usually by Herpes II, was regarded as the most prevalent venereal disease. After an initial skin eruption, the virus hibernates within the nerves supplying the affected area and re-erupts when activated by emotional and physical stress.

Further stressing the patient are the emotional confusion, guilt and feelings of helplessness that can accompany the discomfort and pain of the eruptions. Medical concern has focused primarily on the dangers to an infant delivered from a vaginally infected mother. The possibility of brain damage, blindness or even death in such cases is a valid medical indication for delivery by Caesarian section; these indications apply equally well to maternal Cytomegalo virus (CMV) infections that are also members of the Herpes family.

Conventional medicine has previously had little to offer the victims of Herpes except local palliatives, pain-killers and sympathy. Anti-viral agents are generally more virostatic than virocidal; they modify but seldom cure the disease.

Although generally ignored by conventional physicians, the naturopathic approaches of the health movement can be helpful in controlling Herpes. The Herpes virus thrives in the presence of the amino acid Arginine and is inhibited by Lysine. Lysine rich diets, supplemented by Lysine tablets and the avoidance of Arginine rich foods (nuts, cereals and chocolate) have been widely advocated and used. Zinc and Vitamins C and E are also part of the regime. BHT, an antioxidant widely used as a food preservative is also used for its specific antiviral action against Herpes.

Smallpox vaccinations were formerly extensively used for recurrent herpetic lesions. This practice was discarded because of questionable results and occasional disasters when the live virus was used in immunocompromised patients. The discontinuance of vaccination therapy which followed the apparent eradication of Smallpox throughout the world probably averted other disasters in immunosuppressed individuals.

The Germans, who have used high dose proteolytic enzymes as adjunctive cancer therapy, have also had impressive results in treating Herpes Zoster. Their most widely used enzyme combination has the rather unlikely name Wobe Mugos but the FDA

(Food and Drug Administration) does not allow its importation into the United States. This is presumably because it was used as an adjunct to Laetrile, the controversial cancer therapy of the 1970s.

The German enzymatic treatment of Herpes Zoster was paralleled in this country by the wide use of Protamide, a denatured proteolytic enzyme. Despite its wide popularity among physicians treating Herpes Zoster, and numerous reports of its success, published in proper medical journals, the FDA succeeded in driving it from the market in the 1970s.*

The demise of Protamide also coincided with the FDA's elimination of many non-specific bacterial vaccines from availability. Their safety had never been questioned and their effectiveness had been widely affirmed clinically for over seventy five years. They are especially helpful in the control of herpetic infections and in increasing the patient's general resistance to disease. They stimulate the release of Interferon and Interleukon within the body; both of these substances are under investigation for a role in AIDS therapy.

Development of an effective Herpes-derived vaccine has been limited by the carcinogenic potential of either killed or inactivated Herpes virus.

Homeopathic remedies have been reported helpful in influenza and other viral conditions, including Herpes. The remedies can be taken orally or injected into acupuncture meridian points. Vitamin B-12, effective as a reticuloendothelial stimulant, has been used with varying effectiveness in Herpes Zoster as well as in Trigeminal Neuralgia; the latter is a violently painful condition linked at times to a Herpes infection within the trigeminal nerve.

Among the more interesting therapies is that originated by Dr. J.R. Miller of the University of Alabama. Using progressively

---

*page 51

diluted skin test doses of Influenza vaccine to determine the proper dosage, he has pioneered a desensitizing (?) method of treating both Influenza and other viral conditions, including Herpes. Technically exquisite because of the infinitesimal dosage used, the method is startingly and rapidly effective against the pains and disabilities of even acute Herpes Zoster. Dr. Miller's work has been quietly confirmed and used by other physicians.

The Miller therapy is regarded askance by many physicians and researchers who cannot fit the results into a scientifically valid explanation. They are confused by the homeopathic range of the dilutions used, and Homeopathy is outside scientific respectability. That the procedure has been used by physicians of good repute will probably help it survive obliteration by the FDA.

A relationship of all members of the Herpes family (Herpes I, II, III, Cytomegalovirus and Epstein Barr-virus) with the atherosclerotic process (hardening of the arteries) is considered possible. Traces of these viruses have been found in smooth muscle cells of the vascular system, consistent with the arteriosclerotic lesions found in chickens with Marek's disease (a leukemia-like condition caused by a member of the Herpes family). Some investigators have maintained that arteriosclerotic lesions are a form of benign tumor, stemming from the ability of the Herpes viruses to initiate cell proliferation. As Herpes viruses can exist secluded in body tissues, capable of reactivation without clinical evidence of disease or infectivity, they hang like the sword of Damocles over many unwitting hosts.

Epstein-Barr virus (EBV), recognized as the cause of infectious mononucleosis, is also found in Chinese nasopharyngeal cancer and Burkett's lymphoma, and with Cytomegalovirus is implicated in the AIDS picture. It grows within the epithelium of the throat, and is primarily transmitted by saliva. Almost all adults are presumed to harbor the E-B virus, probably in an inactive form; it can be isolated in twenty percent of healthy asymptomatic adults but from a hundred percent of those who are immunocompromised.

The primary target of the E-B virus is the human B-lymphocyte, which it can "transform" so that when cultured, the "B" lymphocyte is capable of infinite cell divisions; this contrasts with the usually limited number of cell divisions for the cells of each species. Within the body the EBV-stimulates plasma cells (derived from B-lymphocytes) to produce a variety of antibodies; these include antibodies that can react against tissue cells of the body to produce a wide spectrum of autoimmune disease. They can also combine with antigens (reactive substances often of microbial origin) to produce antigen-antibody complexes capable of inducing baffling dysfunctions of many body systems and organs. Lymphocytes "transformed" by the EB virus can produce the uncontrolled cell proliferation from which leukemias and lymphomas develop. This caused the death of David, the well known and beloved "Bubble Boy".

Suppressor T-lymphocytes, increased in an effort to shut down the excess B-cell proliferation, are recognizable in blood smears as the atypical lymphocytes that are diagnostic of infectious mononucleosis.

In 1948, Dr. Raphael Isaacs noted the existence of a chronic syndrome that, following infectious mononucleosis, consisted of chronic fatigue, lethergy, malaise, swollen lymph nodes, and non-specific laboratory findings. There was no great medical interest directed to the condition and the unfortunates who were afflicted with it were usually assigned to the "psychoneurotic" trash basket. This picture has recently emerged to attention again as chronic, relapsing and persistent E-B infection. It is probable that this condition relates to many of the non-specific manifestations of AIDS, particularly of AIDS Related Complex and Opportunistic Infection.

Latent Cytomegalovirus (CMV), like others of the Herpes family, can often emerge to damage or destroy the newborn infant or the immunocompromised adult. It causes more congenital disease than Rubella (German Measles), producing abortion, stillbirth, hepatitis and a wide assortment of baffling neurologic disorders of the newborn. Like the E-B virus, it can produce a mononucleosis-like picture of enlarged lymph nodes, and evidence of systemic disease. CMV antibodies can be demonstrated in fifty percent of the general population and in ninety percent of homosexual males.

CMV's highly variable course in immunocompromised patients can produce fever, pneumonia, leukopenia (low white cell count), brain and eye involvements and an increased incidence of bacterial, protozoal and fungal superinfections of the gastro-intestinal tract and the kidneys. These are prominent features of many AIDS patients, particularly those with Opportunistic Infections.

They are also characteristic of the serious post-operative problems of kidney transplants and open heart surgery. Generally considered to be the reactivation of dormant CMV within the patient, they are likely to come from the accompanying blood transfusions, which, when accompanied by the AIDS Virus can progress to AIDS. An underlying Cytomegalovirus infection is believed to be a factor in preparing the lungs on which Pneumocystis Carinii, the major Opportunistic Infection, develops.

CMV is no longer believed to be the cause of AIDS although its involvements confuse the picture. There is no satisfactory treatment for CMV, so its diagnosis is generally of more academic interest than therapeutic specificity. In kidney transplants, alpha-Interferon reduces the signs of Cytomegalovirus infection and the incidence of Opportunistic infections, although the CMV infection is not eliminated.

These viral infections blend with still other micro-organisms to produce the infinitely variable and confusing picture of AIDS.

Reprinted from the A. M. A. Archives of Ophthalmology
September 1959, Vol. 62, pp. 381-385
Copyright 1959, by American Medical Association

[T]he Treatment of Ophthalmic Herpes Zoster with [P]rotamide

[S]CASSELLATI SFORZOLINI, M.D., Bologna, Italy

[C]linical Evaluation of Protamide in Sensory Nerve Root Inflammations and Allied Conditions

NORTHWEST MEDICINE, NOVEMBER, 1955 **1249**

HENRY W. LEHRER, M.D., HENRY G. LEHRER, M.D., AND DAVID R. LEHRER, M.D.
SANDUSKY, OHIO

HERPES ZOSTER: ITS TREATMENT WITH PROTAMIDE*

FRANK C. COMBS, M. D., and ORLANDO CANIZARES, M. D., NEW YORK CITY

(From the Department of Dermatology and Syphilology of the New York University Post-Graduate Medical School and the Service of Dermatology and Syphilology of Bellevue Hospital)

Reprinted from New York State Journal of Medicine
pp. 706 - 708 (March 15,) 1952

Treatment of Herpes Zoster With Protamide

WILLIAM C. MARSH, *Commander (MC) U. S. N.*[1]

[1] U. S. Naval Hospital, National Naval Medical Center, Bethesda, Md.

1045

Reprinted from U. S. Armed Forces Medical Journal 1:1045 (Sept.) 1950. Protamide is trademark of Sherman Laboratories, Detroit, Mich.

Reprinted From
THE WEST VIRGINIA MEDICAL JOURNAL
(Pages 191-193)
Vol. 56 JUNE, 1960 No. 6

TREATMENT OF HERPES ZOSTER OPHTHALMICUS
(With Case Reports)

By Edward Shupala, M. D.
1052 Market Street
Parkersburg, W. Va.

OPHTHALMIC herpes zoster is characterized by vesicular lesions distributed along the course of the ophthal...

...The mode of action of Protamide, a denatured prote... ic enzyme processed from the glandular layer of the hog's stomach, is still unexplained. The common history of some type of virus infection antedating the neuritis by one to three weeks suggests that this compound is able to exert an antiviral effect upon the infection of the posterior nerve roots, similar to its action in herpes zoster. It is of no value in spinal root syndromes due to mechanical causes.

Reprinted from:
THE MEDICAL CLINICS OF NORTH AMERICA, MARCH, 1957
PUBLISHED BY: W. B. SAUNDERS COMPANY
Philadelphia, Pennsylvania

Reprinted from NEW YORK MEDICINE
pp. 16-17, 18-19 (August 20,) 1952

...ment of Neuritis with Protamide

Richard T. Smith, M.D.†

12

OTHER INFECTIONS OF AIDS

CHLAMYDIAL INFECTIONS are the most prevalent sexually transmitted group of diseases today and yet they have been ignored for any relevance to AIDS.

In addition to Lymphogranuloma Venerum (one of the less common venereal lesions of the skin and lymphatics) they cause Trachoma (a major cause of blindness in parts of Africa) and Psittacosis (Parrot Fever). The Chlamydia family were originally thought to be viruses because of their small size and intracellular life cycles within body tissues; they are now recognized as very small bacteria, composed of both RNA and DNA, unlike viruses which have one but never both of these substances.

Chlamydia produce primarily genital tract infections in adults (generally non-specific urethritis in men and pelvic inflammations in women). Infants delivered from infected women suffer from eye infections, pneumonia and an increased incidence of ear infections and diarrhea in the first year of life.

Despite its wide prevalence, clinicians have ignored a possible role for Chlamydia in the AIDS picture although wide lymphatic involvements are a feature of both inflammatory Kaposi's sarcoma and Chlamydial infections. In 1973, an unusual case was reported of a young male whose overwhelming and fatal Chlamydial infection was manifest by extensive lymphatic involvement throughout his body. He had edema (swelling of the tissues) leukopenia (low white blood cell count) and disseminated Kaposi's sarcoma.* Today, this case would be considered a florid case of AIDS.

CANDIDA ALBICANS, a yeast whose infections are known as Monilia (and popularly as Thrush) is present as a diagnostically suggestive lesser infection of the skin and mucous membranes in almost all cases of AIDS. As the cause of esophagitis, which presents as pain and difficulty in swallowing, it can be diagnostically considered a major opportunistic infection.

Candida's normally controlled existence on skin, mucous membranes and in the bowel can be compromised by immuno-efficiency states. These can be induced by diabetes, pregnancy or the use of certain drugs. Most commonly these are antibiotics, steroids, or birth control pills. "Thrush" is frequently found in the mouths of infants before the full development of their immune systems.

In recent years, chronic and often imperceptible Candida infections have been recognized as associated with severe symptoms referable to every system of the body. Within the intestines, ecologically disturbed from antibiotics, acid-base imbalances or nutritional deficiencies, normally innocuous yeast cells can lose their protective cell walls and develop fungus-like appearances and characteristics. These, invading and functionally distorting the intestinal wall with root-like mycelia, allow multiple antigenic and toxic substances to enter the blood stream and disperse throughout the body.

These substances can affect almost all systems and organs. Although Candida infection cannot be "proved" to be the cause of many poorly defined syndromes, the latter often improve or clear when Candida infections are adequately treated. Favorable results have been reported in autoimmune conditions, neurologic

*page 57

states (multiple sclerosis), gastro-intestinal conditions (Crohn's disease), psychiatric ailments (depression and even schizophrenia) vascular disorders (fluid retention and vasculitis), arthritis, and many poorly treatable environmental and food allergies have also been benefited. It is likely that the immunosuppressive capabilities of Candida may play a role in the evolution of AIDS.

The presence of Candida can increase the toxicity of Staphylococcal infection by multiples of 100,000. This suggests that Candida may be involved with Staphylococci in the production of the Toxic Shock Syndrome. (This, one of the medical mysteries of the 1970s with multiple unexplained deaths, was finally traced to Staphylococcal infections). An occasionally hypersensitive skin reaction to Staphylococcal antigen in AIDS patients is likely due to the synergistic effect of Candida.

Candida infection can cause severe aberrations of T and B lymphocytes with T4/T8 ratio reversals which return to normal when the infection is cleared.

Optimal treatment of Candidal infection involves orthodox antifungal therapy and nutritional regimes. Restoration of normal bowel flora helps to overcome the fungus-like infiltration of Candida within the the bowel walls, thereby helping a return of normal intestinal function. This appears to be as pertinent to the Candida of AIDS as to non-AIDS Candidal infection.

Credit for originating and disseminating Candida's wide role in clinical medicine belongs to Dr. Orion Truss, allergist and internist of Birmingham, Alabama. Dr. Truss has demonstrated the power of the individual to influence medical thought and practice in an era of conformity and regulation. An increasing number of conferences based on yeast interactions have provided a common ground for researchers and clinicians from both scientific and health-oriented areas of medicine.

Body defenses against Chlamydia, as well as Candida, are mainly by T-lymphocytes but these organisms are also ingested and destroyed by the polymorphonuclear white cells (granulocytes) and the macrophages. Under the influence of certain antibiotics and physical agents, Chlamydia, like Candida and many other bacteria, can lose their cell walls and transform into cell wall deficient forms, also known as "pleomorphic" or "L" organisms.* This wide and baffling assortment of micro-organisms, although poorly recognized and accepted in orthodox biologic circles, has bewitched and bedeviled microbiologists since the time of Pasteur. Found as harmless saprophytes in all healthy individuals, their repeated isolation from many disease states suggests more than the casual and harmless relationships that conventional medicine has ascribed to them.

MYCOBACTERIA, the widely spread family to which human, bovine and avian Tuberculosis belong, has cell wall deficient forms. Tuberculosis has come under control and the death rate reduced but there is still a high incidence of infection, mostly unreported, in the United States. Despite many effective therapies, Tuberculosis is incurable; a small number of inactive organisms persist in the body and produce active disease when body defenses are lowered. In under developed countries, Tuberculosis and Leprosy (also caused by a Mycobacterium) are widespread. By themselves or in combination with other diseases, they produce an appalling incidence of illness and death.

Mycobacteria produce assorted diseases in animals, but except for Tuberculosis and Leprosy, their role in human disease has not been generally accepted. Their presence has long been demonstrated in an assortment of diseases, which include Hodgkins Disease, cancer and collagen disease. Recently, Mycobacteria have been fairly conclusively demonstrated to cause Crohn's Disease, a bowel inflammation that has features resembling those found in some cases of AIDS. Dr. Alan Cantwell

---

*Chapter 19.

is a convincing proponent for Mycobacteria's part in the evolution of KAPOSI'S sarcoma.

It is tempting to speculate that a combination of Chlamydia and Mycobacteria might relate to the aggressive form of Kaposi's sarcoma that in this country and Africa is associated with AIDS.

As Chlamydia, Candida and Mycobacteria depress body defenses, their presence, added to parasites and viral infections, undoubtedly plays a large role in the total AIDS picture.

AIDS in 1968

To the Editor.—The recent epidemic of acquired immune deficiency syndrome (AIDS), first reported in 1981,[1] has greatly alarmed the general public. Back in 1973, however, we described in detail[2] a curious clinical syndrome in a native-born American first seen by us in 1968 who in retrospect fulfilled the diagnostic criteria for AIDS.

Report of a Case.—A 15-year-old black male, born and raised in St Louis and who to our knowledge had never left that area, had brawny penile and scrotal edema of one year's duration followed later by bilateral leg edema. He had not previously been seriously ill and specifically had never received a blood transfusion. While he admitted to heterosexual relations for several years, a homosexual history was not specifically elicited. Bilateral pedal lymphangiography revealed complete lymphatic obstruction at the inguinal ligaments with dermal backflow, and an excised inguinal lymph node showed marked fibrosis. Lymphedema was unremitting, and subsequent biopsy of a supraclavicular lymph node showed on light microscopy chronic granulomatous lymphadenitis with fibrosis and disappearance of germinal centers. Over the ensuing 15 months, his clinical course was inexorably downhill, with progressive bilateral pleural effusions, ascites, and anasarca. During an intermittently febrile course, chlamydial microorganisms were repeatedly isolated from blood and body fluids, and hypoproteinemia and peripheral lymphopenia (≈500 to 1,000/cu mm) progressively worsened despite an extended course of antimicrobial therapy including tetracycline, penicillin, sulfisoxazole, and cephalothin sodium. Antibodies to Epstein-Barr virus (EBV) by ox-cell hemolysin and cytomegalovirus (CMV) by complement fixation were undetectable, and both Frei and intermediate PPD skin test results were negative. At autopsy, not only was a cutaneous nodule of Kaposi's sarcoma visible on the medial aspect of the right thigh, but much of the soft tissue throughout the body, including the anorectum, was infiltrated with an angiosarcoma variously interpreted as Kaposi's sarcoma or lymphangiosarcoma. While the rest of the digestive tract was spared, lymph nodes, spleen, and bone marrow exhibited profound lymphocyte depletion with few precursors and extensive fibrosis. The thymus gland showed lymphocyte replacement with plasma cell clusters, absence of Hassall's corpuscles, and also diffuse Kaposi's sarcoma.

Edited by John D. Archer, MD, Senior Editor.

Specimens of plasma and thoracic duct lymph, collected during his lifetime and frozen for 15 years, were thawed earlier this year and restudied. Immunoglobulin G, A, and M levels in these fluids were normal. Serum antibodies were positive by enzyme-linked immunosorbent assay to herpes simplex (1:6,400), rubella (1:3,200), and CMV (1:800); were undetectable to streptolysin O and *Chlamydia trachomatis* (immunofluorescence); and were consistent with past infection to EBV (immunofluorescence).

Comment.—The evolution of this sexually active teenage boy's disease—progression of lymph nodal pathology, fulminant clinical course associated with widespread chlamydial infection, and rapid demise with disseminated Kaposi's sarcoma—makes AIDS a compelling diagnosis in retrospect. Whether chlamydial infection, commonly found in homosexuals, is an etiologic or opportunistic process in AIDS is unresolved, but its ubiquity is nonetheless highly characteristic of the AIDS population. Involvement of the anorectum with obliterative lymphangitis, prominent hemorrhoids, and Kaposi's sarcoma with concomitant sparing of the remainder of the gastrointestinal tract suggests the rectum as the portal of entry for chlamydia, as oftentimes is the case in the closely related syndrome of lymphopathia venereum. Of interest, this latter disorder may also display brawny penile and scrotal edema, fibrotic inguinal lymphadenitis, and peripheral lymphedema.

Although some claim that AIDS is newly imported to the continental United States, the typical features exemplified by our native-born American patient suggest that the syndrome is, at least in part, endemic and appeared more than ten years before the current epidemic.

MARLYS H. WITTE, MD
CHARLES L. WITTE, MD
LINDA L. MINNICH, MS
PAUL R. FINLEY, MD
University of Arizona
College of Medicine
Tucson
WILLIAM L. DRAKE, JR, MD
Missouri Baptist and
Deaconess Hospitals
St Louis

1. Curran JW: AIDS: Two years later. *N Engl J Med* 1983;309:609-610.
2. Elvin-Lewis M, Witte M, Witte C, et al: Systemic chlamydial infection associated with generalized lymphedema and lymphangiosarcoma. *Lymphology* 1973;6:113-121.

13

DIMENSIONS OF ENERGY

In 1971, James Reston, while reporting from China on the resumption of Sino-American relations, had his appendix removed under acupuncture anesthesia. His widely published account of the operation made acupuncture a household word and brought it to the attention of Western medicine, which has accepted it as a generally inexplicable form of analgesia; Western culture has only lightly approached the philosophy and practices of Chinese medicine which underlie its efffectiveness for many conditions.

For several thousand years, the Chinese have charted the flow of energy over and through the body by meridian-aligned points; they consider imbalance or blockage of this flow to produce disturbed physio-chemical function, and eventually, organic disease. In the philosophy and medicine of India, vortices of energy termed "chakras" are thought to complement the energy meridians of Oriental medicine and correspond closely to the neuro-humoral influences of our major endocrine glands. Many theoreticians believe that the subtle remedies of Homeopathy achieve their effects through energy realignments, and it may be that the successes of Chiropractic and classic Osteopathy have more to do with unblocking the flow of energy than with straightening out anatomic problems.

Public expectations that acupuncture would prove a medical panacea have not been realized although the demonstration that acupuncture can trigger a release of endorphins (chemicals capable of influencing pain and other sensory perceptions) from the brain has provided acceptably scientific grounds for considering acupuncture a medical adjunct. By its nature, acupuncture is incapable of the proof of efficacy requirements of Scientific Medicine.

Acupuncture aligns with biofeedback, the placebo effect, visualization therapy, healing techniques and the role of attitudes and emotions in health and illness.

Western science has been somewhat prepared for energy concepts in a larger setting by the lifelong researches of the late Dr. Harold Saxon Burr of Yale Medical School. Using a microvoltage meter capable of measuring infinitely small gradations in an energy field without abstracting energy or disrupting the field under study, he demonstrated that all forms of life are controlled by electrodynamic forces which he called "L" or life fields; these can be mapped with great precision, and confirm that each system of life is embedded through its own electrodynamic field in its immediate environment as well as in the electromagnetic fields of earth and in radiations from space.

Burr's work connects Western technology to Eastern concepts of universal energy as the central force in the growth and development of all living matter. It helps to provide a rationale for acupuncture, Kirlian photography, Homeopathy, electromagnetic healing, negative ions, polarity therapy, Yoga, Chiropractic and other approaches. These, long outside the province of Scientific Medicine, are incorporated in what is termed "holistic" medicine.

The term "holistic" is difficult to define. The dictionary defines holism as "the philosophic theory that whole entities, as fundamental and determining components of reality, have an existence other than as the mere sum of its parts". This originally precise definition has been warped by indiscriminate usage. For many, it has become a synonym for "open minded and progressive" with the positive connotation that "natural" carries for many people. Many practitioners and organizations describe themselves as "holistic" when "health oriented" would be more accurate.

Holism is a multi-disciplinary movement that considers health and medicine as aspects of the ultimate integration of the individual with all aspects of existence and of his surroundings. Genuinely holistic practitioners seek the total integration of mind and body through nutrition, exercise, self-regulatory techniques such as biofeedback, meditation, neuromuscular manipulations, acupuncture and hypnosis. They also use conventional medical therapy as needed. Holism aligns with the concept of mind as manifesting a central, all permeating energy which creates and defines reality for the individual.

Only recently has medicine recognized its roots in the relationships of mind, body and spirit, which have been inextricably bound together in tribal cultures and primitive societies. The Greeks displaced illness and disease from the realm of the supernatural; their naturopathic orientation was expressed by "Vis Medicatrix Naturae" (the healing force of Nature). This emphasized the ability of the body to heal itself when environmental conditions of pure food and water, fresh air and mental equilibrium, are achieved. This recurrent eddy in the medical mainstream is evident as health-oriented concepts today.

The Renaissance released Western man from medieval concepts of illness and disease as trials or punishments from God. Rationalism, based on the Cartesian concept of the body as a superb machine governed by physical and chemical laws, was the basis for the subsequent development of Scientific Medicine. This mechanistic orientation had its counterbalance in Vitalism, which holds that a self-determining, self-evolving energy, distinct from physical and chemical forces, underlies all manifestations of life.

Average physicians, practicing Scientific Medicine to the degree that average Christians follow the precepts of Christ, have little time for Health Oriented Medicine; they generally classify holistic concepts with the social sciences, which are also poorly measured or evaluated. Concepts of mind and spirit are lumped with religion or philosophy and considered important only if they help the patient adjust psychologically to his circumstances. However, they are essential in any approach to AIDS.

It is not always easy to deal with AIDS patients, and particularly when they have Opportunistic Infection. As a generalization, they are creative, sensitive, attractive and emotionally labile individuals who react poorly to the demands and responsibilities of any illness. When confronted with the diagnosis of AIDS, they are often shattered and poorly capable of involvement in their own treatment or care. Like many cancer patients, they have difficulty in expressing anger, in fighting, or in adjusting to stress; the poorest survival rates and highest recurrences in both conditions are among those overcome by depression, helplessness and hopelessness. Workers have commented on the inner awareness beneath the depressions and self destructive urges that are in the background of many AIDS patients. Their conflicts and inner turmoil are often obscured or displaced by the anxiety, depression and resignation that accompany the diagnosis of AIDS.

The decreased ability of many AIDS patients to function well for themselves often has an organic as well as a psychologic basis. The AIDS virus, in addition to its effects on the cells of the immune system, appears to have a predilection for nerve cells. It produces encephalopathy and impaired cerebral function in many patients, as well as peripheral nerve involvements in others. The psychologic and neurologic malfunctions caused by the AIDS virus cannot be easily distinguished from those caused by other co-existing viruses such as Cytomegalovirus or the Herpes virus. Tumors of the nervous tissue (most frequently lymphomas) are still another diagnostic and therapeutic problem in these patients.

Western culture has lacked a unified concept of spirit, mind and body. There is, however, an increasing awareness that spiritual considerations, beyond intellect or emotions, and unconfined to religion or creed, are basic to all aspects of life, extending beyond the burdens of illness and disease.

Spiritual aspects, apart from the emotional and intellectual composition of the individual AIDS patient, are difficult to comprehend or consciously recognize. They are a large factor, however, in the relatively good outlook for those with AIDS Related Complex or Kaposi's sarcoma alone, compared to those who develop Opportunistic Infection. When their body defenses are strained but not overwhelmed, many (approximately eighty percent) of the former can contain their illness or slowly improve. By improving or changing their life styles, their nutrition, their environment and their inner "life awareness", they enable their bodies to maintain the status quo or begin the long, slow, healing process.

It is an evolvement from self-centeredness to a broader concept of identity and life purpose that separates the successfully controlled AIDS patient from those who go steadily downhill. They achieve the dimensions of those covered by Frankl in "The Unheeded Cry for Meaning":

"Being human is being always directed, and pointing, to something or someone other than oneself; to a meaning to fulfill or another human being to encounter, a cause to serve or a person to love. Only to the extent that someone is living out this self-transcendence of human existence, is he truly human or does he become his true self. He becomes so, not by concerning himself with his self's actualization, but by forgetting himself and giving himself, overlooking himself and focusing outward. . . . What is called self-actualization, is and must remain, the unintended effect of self transcendence; it is ruinous and self defeating to make it the target of intention. And what is true of self actualization also holds for identity and happiness. It is the very pursuit of happiness that obviates happiness."

A SPIRITUAL READING OF AIDS

All things of the human body are simply communication. The emergence of AIDS indicates that there is a new language that has emerged into the physical realm. The properties inherent in its physical manifestations are the ability to manifest deep spiritual needs and emotional reactions. AIDS is a language which, once understood (decoded), is no longer the mystery the enigma, it has presented till now. It is simply another language of the body that is speaking the words which consciousness has deemed itself unable to speak, and yet the unspeakable must be spoken, the unseeable must be envisioned, the unthinkable, thought. In other words, those who are crippled, diseased, and in extreme terror are those who hold within themselves, without exceptions, areas of fear which must speak through the powers of such a debilitating illness. They must allow themselves to move into areas of spirituality and into the deeper processes of understanding the purpose of life and respect of all things in human life. All things must be seen and acknowledged before they can be transformed. Healing can take place, and what may seem miraculous healing, if the voice of the soul, the language of the illness, can be understood. The willingness to hear ones own inner voice is tantamount to beginning the healing process. Again, the unthinkable must be thought and nothing is unthinkable but the judgements and the self punishment of those who are experiencing such an anguishing deterioration.

by: Emmanuel

14

CANCER AND AIDS

Cancer and AIDS have strong parallels. They are currently the cause and the symptoms of our greatest social and personal miseries, their causes have not been unequivocally determined, and their treatments are generally unsatisfactory. The evolution of both conditions relate to nutrition, environment, life styles and stress. The recent interest of cancer researchers in prevention and in aspects of health relating to nutrition, life styles and the effects of stress upon the body's defense mechanisms, has not yet been equalled by those working in the AIDS field.

The current assault by medical researchers against AIDS has followed the well funded and much heralded War Against Cancer, begun in the 1970s. Both have been largely dominated by the search for the viral cause and the chemical cure of their respective conditions. Recognition that pleomorphic organisms participate in AIDS might also direct attention to their role in cancer. The virus-like spore stage of pleomorphic organisms may be among the long sought viral causes of cancer and other degenerative disease.

It has been noted that the late stages of cancer and AIDS are often indistinguishable. Pertinent to AIDS is Dr. Max Gerson's summation that: "Cancer is a chronic degenerative disease where almost all essential organs are involved in the more advanced cases; the entire metabolism, with the intestinal tract and its adnexa, the liver and pancreas, the circulatory apparatus, the kidneys and bile system, the reticuloendothelial and lymphatic system, the central nervous system and especially the visceral nervous system for most metabolic purposes".

Cancers (and particularly lymphomas and squamous cell carcinoma of the skin) are intimately associated with AIDS. It has been suggested that these occuring on the head and neck of those at risk of AIDS, should automatically be classified as AIDS. Homosexual males have an increased rate of rectal cancer.

It has been shown that the malignancy rate of patients with primary immunodeficiency is one hundred times that of controls, with lymphomas (malignancies of the lymphatic and connective tissue) being the most prominent.

Research has suggested that much cancer might be initiated by innocuous-appearing infections, with the Herpes family prominent among the suspects. A Johns Hopkins study has demonstrated that women who marry men whose former wives died of cervical cancer develop cancer of the cervix at four times the normal incidence of the disease. This suggests the male as an unwitting accessory to his wife's cancer. The wives of men who have prostatic cancer have also been found to have an elevated rate of gynecologic cancer. Current studies have also indicated a relationship of uterine cancer to prior herpetic genital infections; other studies have suggested that herpetic viruses might be related to much head and neck cancer.

Cancer has traditionally been considered an uncontrolled tissue growth which originates in a single cell and spreads to overwhelm the body with its parasitic overgrowths. This conception of a malign autonomous process has dominated medical thinking so that classic therapy has been largely surgical, seeking early recognition and complete extirpation of the tumor before its roots have penetrated and its tendrils have spread. In the

United States, this philosophy has been the basis for the popularity among surgeons of radical mastectomy for breast cancer despite the physical and psychic mutilation of the patient.

Low dose X-rays, deriving from the classic animal work of Murphy at Rockefeller Institute seventy years ago, were originally used to stimulate local tissue resistance against cancer. Improved radiation technology made possible the selective destruction of cancer cells, with radiation dosage limited only by damage to adjacent tissues. After World War II, cancer therapy followed this silver bullet concept with the development of selective chemicals to poison the cancer cell. The therapeutic specificity of surgery, radiation and chemotherapy has been counterbalanced by their toxic and often delayed side effects; these have obscured the evidence that cancer is essentially a chronic disesase. It appears that our modes of life and our therapies by depleting our body defenses often transform our cancers into rapidly progressive disease. This parallels the current treatment of AIDS-related Kaposi's sarcoma; the lesions may variably regress, but the condition of the patient often progresses to Opportunistic Infection.

In 1969 there was much perplexity when Dr Hardin Jones, a reputable statistician at the University of Califonia, reported that statistically the life expectancy of cancer patients is greater without treatment. This remarkable conclusion is probably explained by the depression of our reticuloendothelial systems from well meant but imperceptive use of therapeutic technology; we have used meat cleavers instead of dissection knives. It may be that Ivan Illich's thesis of the illness-producing capability of modern medicine is best illustrated in the cancer field.

The immunologic concept of cancer therapy has had a long and slow development. Most clinicians, long dominated by the surgical tradition, are reluctant to accept or use the concept that the healing capacity of the body, as well as its resistance to cancer, can be augmented. There have recently been some encouraging results from specific tumor vaccines. The use of non-specific bacterial vaccines to increase body resistance is again being recognized although vaccines and serums derived from microorganisms have long been prominent in the unorthodox therapies denied by the American Cancer Society and vigorously prosecuted by the Food and Drug Administration.

When body defenses are good, virulent organisms are more easily overcome by the judicious use of antibiotics. Chemotherapy and radiotherapy in the treatment of cancer, and antiviral agents in the treatment of AIDS are also more effective when body defenses are good. The overuse and misuse of the chemotherapy and radiation in cancer are comparable to the overuse and misuse of antibiotics in medicine. Someday, they will be viewed as we now view the treatment of war wounds before Pare' (The 15th century French surgeon whose humane treatment of injuries abolished the use of boiling oil that had previously been standard therapy) or the late 18th century practice of bleeding and purging terminally ill patients.

The pressures that weigh on clinical oncologists apply to those who care for AIDS patients; they must satisfy their own emotional needs and motivations while trying to cope with the fears and anxieties of patients and their families and the narrow range of alternatives available when therapy is ineffective. Too often, the physician is encased in a layer of objectivity and detachment, essential for his own psychic survival but poorly oriented to the needs of patients and their families. Too many clinicians, focused only on the therapeutic tightrope they tread, do not appreciate that the body defense systems and the patient's own motivations influence the long term therapy of cancer or AIDS.

Successful clinicians encourage and support their patients with therapeutic regimes that are understandable and acceptable to them. Aware of their patient's emotional, mental and spiritual capacities, they utilize them therapeutically. The personality profiles of the cancer patient as outlined by LeShan and others, and the demonstration by the Simontons of the healing capacities inherent in every patient, are especially pertinent. Also relevant to AIDS is Michio Kushi's observation that for many patients, life is a disease and cancer is one of its cures. The final breakdown into cancer is precipitated, but not caused, by unrelated but cumulative factors, such as loneliness, grief and depression. These same factors have been noted to be operative in AIDS by researchers of psycho-immunology, the newest investigative discipline, that includes all aspects of psychologic factors and their direct effects on the immune system.

Patients who survive cancer or AIDS, regardless of therapy, invariably possess inner reserves by which they re-order their lives and their priorities. Too often, patients do not want to die or suffer but they have no compelling purpose for living; they submit passively to regimes and procedures to please their families or their physician and they spiral uncomplainingly downward. The litmus question to a cancer or AIDS patient "What real reason do you have for living?" is often unanswerable. The will to live must come from the patient and no amount of anguish, encouragement or entreaties from family or friends will help if this is not present.

Search for a universal cancer or AIDS cure has obscured recognition that they will recur when their predisposing conditions remain. We can aim for reasonable control with multiple therapies, much as we can control most infections with antibiotics, but the surest therapy is prevention. By improving our environment, our life styles and our deeper motivations, we can help to resist the stresses that we impose, or allow to be imposed, on our bodies.

15

ADJUNCTIVE AIDS THERAPY

As with cancer, the background factors that influence the progression of the individual AIDS patient belong more to the health movement than to the medical profession. These include motivation, life style, emotional and spiritual values, proper nutrition and environment. In urban areas, where AIDS is most often found, the ancient Greek precepts of proper diet, fresh air, pure water, sunshine and inner serenity are difficult, if not impossible, for the majority of AIDS patients to achieve.

AIDS patients who have achieved control of their disease are seldom found in the clinics and programs of research centers from which reports and official statistics on AIDS originate. These patients usually attend private physicians who cooperate with them in exploring avenues of reasonable therapy and who treat all aspects of their disease.

These patients investigate, ask questions and are informed on all aspects of AIDS. They develop an awareness of themselves, often patronize health food stores and read health-oriented publications. Some use acupuncturists, naturopaths, nutritionists, homeopaths, and healers and they are as sceptical and selective of these as they are of conventional practitioners and orthodox therapy. They select those with whom they feel comfortable and they work with them and share responsibility in their treatments. Almost without exception, they develop and draw on spiritual resources and alignments from within themselves.

So far, there has been no diagnostic test for the immunosuppression that is central to the onset of AIDS. It is possible that the modified lipid-bound sialic acid (LASA) test, developed at Sloan Kettering Institute by Drs. Katapodis and Stock as a non-specific index of cancer activity, might be also pertinent to AIDS. Lipid bound sialic acid levels have been reported low in early pregnancy, gradually increasing to normal levels at delivery time. Patients with AIDS have also been found to have levels appreciably below the normal range of values. While research with this test has been primarily limited to cancer, it may be a handle for evaluating those at risk of AIDS as well as for monitoring those under treatment.

Non-specific bacterial vaccines honorably used in Europe, and until recently in this country, for many chronic conditions, are now recognized to function as reticuloendothelial stimulants. Coley's Toxins, now known as Mixed Bacterial Toxins (MBT) and belatedly recognized by the Medical Establishment as an effective cancer therapy in certain cases, was also considered to be an effective reticuloendothelial stimulant in a wide variety of degenerative diseases.

Despite wide and empiric usage of bacterial vaccines, amply reported in medical literature since the turn of the century, there has been little recognition within Academia of their value. The advent of antibiotics diminished their usage and the 1960s "proof of efficacy" requirements of the FDA proved too expensive for small companies to comply with, and provided an excuse for the larger companies to cease production of these generally unprofitable items. Their safety had never been questioned and their effectiveness had been attested to by thousands of physicians and patients who had benefited from them. The only non-specific vaccines still available in this country are Staphage Lysate of the Delmont Laboratories* and the Mixed Respiratory Vaccine of the Hollister Stier Company.

Another effective adjunct to general health measures, particularly applicable to the treatment of AIDS, is auto-transfusion of small amounts of the patient's blood which has been irradiated by ultra violet light.* This procedure, known as the Knott technique after the inventor of the equipment, was a small but impeccably documented medical therapy for viral and bacterial infections in the 1930s and 1940s. Its usage died out following the advent of antibiotics but it has been recently revived in Germany, where, with small but technically precise equipment, it is used for an impressive range of medical conditions that range from infection to vascular disorders. The exact manner in which it exerts its beneficial results is not known, although it is considered to stimulate both the reticuloendothelial and the properdin systems of the body. Credit is also given to the ozone produced by the ultra-violet rays reacting with the oxygen that pushes the blood through the equipment.

Ozone therapy, closely related to ultra-violet irradiation of blood, has been extensively used and reported from Europe for the past decade as treatment for infections of all kinds, cancer, and circulatory disturbances. Despite its wide and academic acceptance there, the Medical Establishment in this country considers it unproven, unimportant and controversial. However, an increasing number of physicians are quietly investigating and using ozone generators for the conditions cited above. Its reported effectiveness in helping AIDS patients can be attributed to its oxidizing properties directed against the background infections of the AIDS patient.

Another empiric therapy for infections, also used as adjunctive cancer therapy, from the First World War until the advent of antibiotics, was the intravenous administration of very dilute

---

*Chapter 38

hydrochloric acid. Without affecting the acid-base balances of the blood, it boosts both the number and the activity of granulocytes and phagocytes (those white blood cells whose scavaging activity comprises the phagocytic system of defense). It improves the oxygen carrying capacity of the blood and generally helps many of the same conditions as ultraviolet irradiated blood and ozone. Hydrochloric acid therapy, because of its economy and availability, was widely used in rural areas where the technology and pharmaceuticals of the day were not available. "The Medical World"*, a now defunct medical journal, devoted many articles and editorials to promote the dissemination and evaluation of this therapy, but except for a few pragmatic physicians who still quietly use it, hydrochloric acid therapy is almost unknown today. Its ability to increase the depressed white blood cell count in certain cases might focus attention on its capabilities in other medical areas.

Acupuncture**, a concept until recently foreign to western medicine, has also been used as adjunctive therapy for AIDS with improvements noted in fever, diarrhea, strength and in almost all parameters of the disease. Homeopathy, a controversial aspect of medicine which allies to the stimulation of the natural healing force of the body by the use of infinitely diluted doses of highly energized substances, is also used by some. The rationale for its use makes no sense to conventional "scientific" physicians, who regard it at best as a placebo. While subtle in its action, it is regarded as beneficial in some cases, although it is often inactivated when used with conventional chemical pharmaceuticals.

The concept that much illness originates from disturbed bowel function is a recurrent theme in medicine. Dr. Max Ger-

---

*page 77

**Chapter 32

son**, known for his successful dietary regimes in degenerative disease, was particularly concerned with bowel cleansing as a detoxification measure, as well as a stimulant of liver function. His work has been the basis for many of the health-oriented nutritional regimes of alternative medicine today. Standard among health-oriented AIDS patients are enemas or colonics with bowel cleansing preparations and Lactobacillus preparations to promote growth of normal bowel organisms.

In AIDS and cancer, almost all dietary regimes restrict sugar, alcohol, coffee, salt, red meat, fats, synthetic additives, white flour and almost all processed foods. Despite its hackle-raising effects on orthodox nutritionists, Macrobiotic regimes* have a following among AIDS patients.

Protomorphogens (organ extracts widely used by alternative practitioners and ignored by orthodox physicians) are considered of value in promoting endocrine functions of the glands. These were developed by Dr. Royal Lee, DDS, founder of the Standard Process Laboratories, and a prolific inventor and nutritional researcher of the first half of this century. He strongly advocated natural and not synthetic vitamins and his research in protomorphogens anticipated the role of DNA as the basic determinant for molecular structure. Addressing the problem of infections (which in the 1920s occupied the role in medical consciousness that stress does today), he stated "We have a vicious cycle in which vitamin starvation produces susceptibility to infectious disease, the overworking of the endocrines to fight the disease increases the need for vitamins and the exhaustion of the endocrines increases the susceptibility to infections".

The foregoing from Dr. Lee aligns with the later notation by Hans Selye that "When suitable raw materials (nutrients,

---

*Chapter 35

---

*Chapter 36

minerals, vitamins) are not available from dietary deficiency, chemical interventions, etc., then the ability of the adrenals to respond to stressful stimuli is impaired." This is of particular pertinency to AIDS patients with long standing and debilitating diarrheas and gastro-intestinal dysfunctions.

Amino acids are increasingly used to enhance strength as well as to boost the immune system. Ornithine and Arginine, by stimulating production of the pro-inflammatory growth hormone (STH, somatotrophic hormone) by the pituitary, help to normalize lymphocyte abnormalities, especially the T4T8 ratio imbalances, which are so prominent in AIDS. In severely ill AIDS patients, hyperalimentation (long term intravenous nutritional therapy) has also been noted of value in helping to restore integrity to the immune system. Hormonal and enzymatic deficits and imbalances, present in almost all degenerative disease states, are improved by proper replacement therapy and nutritional supplements of hydrochloric acid, vitamins, minerals, nucleic acids, amino acids and pancreatic enzymes. That Arginine contributes to the growth of the Herpes virus even as it strengthens the T-lymphocytes, emphasizes how little we know of amino acid interactions within the body.

The benefits of ascorbic acid (Vitamin C) in AIDS aligns to orthomolecular medicine. This latter concept by Dr. Linus Pauling is defined as "the achievement and preservation of health by varying those substances that are normally present in the body, such as vitamins". Man, along with the simians and the guinea pig, is unable to synthesize ascorbic acid and must obtain it from food sources, which are usually inadequate. On the basis of comparative animal studies, it has been suggested that our daily intake of ascorbic acid should range from 6 to 20 grams.

The increasing use within Health Oriented Medicine of high dose intravenous ascorbic acid for severe infections is credited to Dr. F.R. Klenner of North Carolina; for over thirty years he has tirelessly advocated and demonstrated that megadoses of intravenous ascorbic acid are effective and safe therapy for resistant bacterial and viral infections.

Dr. Robert Cathcart of California has confirmed and reaffirmed Dr. Klenner's contributions. In all forms of AIDS, he has demonstrated impressive results with massive intravenous ascorbic acid therapy in properly motivated patients. When the patient is stabilized, he is then switched to oral therapy. Ascorbic acid is an integral factor of a comprehensive regime aimed at maximal restoration and maintenance of the patient's natural defenses.

Under normal circumstances, the beneficial effects of adequately oxygenated body tissues cannot be over-emphasized. It enhances metabolism and benefits all aspects of the reticuloendothelial system. It directly aligns with the General Adaptation Syndrome of Selye as a beneficial stress that protects at local levels against otherwise detrimental conditions. In AIDS, however, as in many debilitating conditions, exercise must be carefully adapted to the individual. Exercise relates to the observation of Kaposi patients that the occurence rate of new lesions relates to the amount they exercise. Patients in control of their Kaposi lesions, almost without exception, exercise regularly and have given up smoking.

The frequent emergence of anaerobic organisms (those usually pathogenic microbes that thrive in the absence of oxygen) and wide debilities from anemia make imperative all measures that increase the amount of oxygen and its use by body tissues, These include vitamins B12 and Folic acid, the oxydizing enzymes of Warburg, thyroid administration to increase the usually depressed metabolism, ultra-violet irradiation of blood, and ozone therapy.

Iron medication may be inadvisable in cases of anemia found so often in AIDS, cancer and many infections. Research has demonstrated that iron is a necessary substrate for many pathogenic microbes and for cancer cells. This characterizes many of the organisms found in AIDS and may account for patients' often unexplained low levels of serum iron. Dr. Maria de Sousa*, formerly of Sloan Kettering Institute, is probably the world authority on the relationships of iron and the immune system. That AIDS Related Complex is not classified as AIDS by medical authorities has deprived the latter of observing and learning from the improvements possible with adjunctive therapies.

Patients, especially those with Kaposi's sarcoma alone, or with AIDS Related Complex, can achieve control with alternative therapies when they have motivation, patience and self discipline; these qualities are in short supply and more easily described than developed. The majority of AIDS Patients are looking for an escalator to ride up the mountain; the ones who achieve the top, however, have usually sought the trail and with guidance have climbed it themselves.

---

*Chapter 34

THREE YEARS OF HCl THERAPY

AS RECORDED IN ARTICLES
APPEARING IN

THE MEDICAL WORLD

WITH INTRODUCTION BY

HENRY PLEASANTS, JR., A.B., M.D., F.A.C.P.
Associate Editor

INTRODUCTION

The awakening of interest on the part of the medical profession in the use of dilute hydrochloric acid intravenously, intramuscularly, orally and locally in the treatment of many disease conditions warrants a condensed outline of the principles upon which this therapeutic measure is based; a resume of our own experiences with it in certain cases; a frank discussion of its limitations, and a general outline of its possibilities. The fact that this agent is so inexpensive; that it is not an exploited compound put out by pharmaceutical manufacturers, and that its usefulness was developed by two practicing physicians, working independently along entirely different theoretical lines, brings this remedy into a position of economic importance that should not be disregarded.

CONTENTS

CONTENTS (Continued)

16

LESSONS FROM AIDS

A IDS is a prototype of degenerative disease, condensing in a relatively short period many of its manifestations. It also demonstrates the urgency of our sexual impulses, the frailties of our human nature in dealing with them, and the limits of our collective humanity when treating its victims. It illustrates the inflexibility and narrow focus of Scientific Medicine when faced with the biologic challenges of AIDS.

There are scattered reports of patients who do not fit the usual AIDS picture to justify the ominous forecasts of an increasing incidence of AIDS in all aspects of society. Despite these, it appears that in Western nations AIDS will be confined to those with overloaded, damaged, or inadequate body defenses against the additional assaults of the AIDS virus. The homosexual community and those who use drugs will undoubtedly remain the groups at greatest risk.

A recent and significant medical article reported that the antibody titer in the wife of a hemophiliac AIDS patient declined and disappeared when she was no longer in contact with her husband's spermatic fluid. This aligns to the Scandinavian study showing that healthy immunocompetent homosexuals are resistant to AIDS virus infection, as indicated by antibody titer.

Combined with Stewart's Australian study*, it suggests that although the immunosuppressive capacity of spermatic fluid on mucous membranes may facilitate entrance of the AIDS virus into the recipient of contaminated semen, a healthy individual may contain the infection from pathogenicity or transmission to others, and may even overcome the infection, as manifest by antibody titer.

The vulnerability of mucous membranes, immunosupressed by seminal fluid contact, to fungal infections and malignancy may well underlie the increased incidence of Candida, Kaposi lesions, and malignancies in the oral and gastrointestinal tracts of immunosuppressed homosexuals.

Local immunosuppression by spermatic fluid facilitates the absorption of viral agents into the general circulation but the antibacterial properties of spermatic fluid probably prevent similarly transmitted bacterial infections.

The repeated local immunosuppressant effect of spermatic fluid, accompanied by viral and other pathogens, undoubtedly is a major mechanism resulting from the background promiscuity of patients with sexually transmitted AIDS.

The treatment of Opportunistic Infection, paralleling many other acute diseases, will remain primarily hospital based and within the domain of Scientific Medicine. It will be increasingly viewed as comparable to pre-antibiotic pneumonia whose treatment with type specific pneumococcal serum (considered the ultimate in scientific technology) was only the first step in a long and slow rebuilding of the damaged body.

Agents effective against the individual opportunists, augmented by other substances to reverse the underlying immunodepression, will remain the keystone of therapy. These will be most effective when combined with measures adequate to rebuild

---

*page 28

the defense and metabolic systems eroded in the course of the disease. It is in this area that Scientific Medicine must modify some of its academic arrogance and learn from Health Oriented Medicine, an area it has previously ignored.

AIDS Related Complex and Kaposi's sarcoma (when alone) indicate the body is struggling with serious but often controllable conditions. It suggests the fundamental importance of life style modification, including proper nutrition, the cessation of all recreational drug use, and the proper treatment of the infections that accompany the AIDS virus. Individual responsibility is the keynote of treatment with recognition that mental, emotional and spiritual factors are adjuncts to health principles, environment, and specific therapy.

A re-evaluation by Scientific Medicine of its overuse and misuse of blood and blood products also applies to antibiotics. Long range debilities from both of these therapies must be more fully balanced against their short term value in individual cases. Blood and antibiotics, the most widely recognized triumphs of scientific medicine, are too often used as crutches; they compare to the widespread use in Victorian times of opium for the sedation of infants and as an effective headache remedy.

As we have eliminated and controlled bacterial infections (eg: streptococcal and staphylococcal) our defense mechanisms, mediated mainly through our reticuloendothelial systems, have weakened. Viral infection, an increasingly widespread hazard to health, too often resistant to antibiotics and antiviral agents, can be compared to insects and weeds; these also flourish and resist our most advanced and expensive technologies against them.

Probably the most important lesson, painfully learned and slowly accepted, is that the AIDS virus will be a permanent addition to mankind's roster of pathogenic microbes. Aligning with Cytomegaloviruses and Epstein-Barr viruses, (whom it closely resembles) and the Tubercule bacillus, it can be a harmless inhabitant in healthy individuals but a deadly threat to those with inadequate body defenses. It is the responsibility of the individual to do all in his power to remain healthy and resistant to the progressions of illness that comprise the categories of AIDS.

In the future, the major transmitting source for the AIDS virus to the general public, (and the least amenable to investigation) will be the bisexual segment of the population, not those who are exclusively homosexual. Bisexuals, infected with the AIDS virus from their homosexual activity can transmit it to their wives and other sexual partners, thereby perpetuating the virus among the general population.

The caution with which homosexual males now view each other, and their current awareness of the danger of unprotected and promiscuous sexual activity, is probably equalled by that of unmarried urban females; the latter must now view many eligible and atractive males with suspicion. It is not beyond probability that proof of having had an AIDS antibody determination will be eventually required for all marriage licenses. It is certain, however, that casual sex among all the population will be less prevalent than before the emergence of AIDS.

17

IN THE WINGS

One of the more provocative papers concerning AIDS was published by Drs. Moskowitz, Hensley, Gould and Weiss of the Univ. of Miami Medical School in the May 1985 issue of Human Pathology. It is a meticulous microscopic study of autopsy material from 52 patients who died of AIDS; these included 23 Haitians (17 men and 6 women), 19 homosexual men, four male and one female intravenous drug users, two hemophiliacs, and one man and two women who did not belong to any known risk group.

Although Opportunistic Infection was the major cause of death, Kaposi's sarcoma was found in 49 (94%) of the cases. This rather startling finding exceeds all previous estimates or reported incidence of Kaposi's sarcoma in AIDS. This is in unexplained contrast to statistics from Belle Glade, Florida. Here, no cases of Kaposi's sarcoma has been reported although the incidence of AIDS is the highest in the United States.

The article reports that the classic pattern of non-inflammatory Kaposi's sarcoma was prevalent in homosexual men of the study; it was never found alone, but was always accompanied by inflammatory Kaposi lesions which were also found in all risk groups. The authors, unlike other investigators, feel that classic and inflammatory Kaposi lesions are separate although often co-existing entities and that neither is the pre-cursor of the other. Commenting that the clinical course of their patients often resembled that of an aggressive malignancy, they feel that the inflammatory and classic Kaposi lesions in these patients were equally ominous.

The authors state that they have found a number of cases of Kaposi's sarcoma in presumable pre-AIDS cases (AIDS-Related Complexes?) in which at the time, T-cell counts and ratios were minimally depressed. Parenthetically, they have noted the presence of blood factor VIII related markers and antigen in the blood of pre-AIDS patients (AIDS Related Complex) as well as in AIDS patients at any stage of the disease.

This study, with its in-depth examination of previously unreported and generally unexpected Kaposi lesions, presents findings, patterns and questions that challenge the presumptions of conventional AIDS research. It clearly points the absolute necessity of defining the relationships of Kaposi's sarcoma to that of Opportunistic infection.

Attempts to resolve this enigma will probably bring from the wings to center stage a cast of medical researchers whose contributions, outside the Medical Establishment, are relevant to AIDS.

A fresh focus on Kaposi's sarcoma will suggest a return to the work of Dr. Hans Selye and his Adaptation Syndrome, which pertains to all aspects of AIDS but especially to Kaposi's sarcoma.

Equally pertinent is Dr. Alan Cantwell, a California dermatologist with a long interest in cancer research. His 1984 book "AIDS—The Mystery & the Solution",* anticipating the Moskowitz study's focus on Kaposi's sarcoma, is a comprehensive summary of all facets of the background of AIDS and of Kaposi's sarcoma. Before the eruption of the AIDS epidemic, Dr. Cantwell had worked in the uncrowded field of pleomorphic

---

*published by: Aries Rising Press Box 29532, Los Angeles, CA 90029

(cell wall deficient) organisms and their relevance to disease, particularly cancer. In 1981, he presented the first of his papers on the presence of these organisms, and particularly Mycobacteria, in Kaposi lesions, but this was little noted or regarded. In his book, Dr. Cantwell documents the large and generally neglected evidence for the role of non-viral microorganisms in cancer and now in AIDS. Other reports implicating Mycobacteria in Kaposi's sarcoma, and in all forms of AIDS, combine with Dr. Moskowitz's findings to encourage fresh attention to this area.

The microscope of Gaston Naessens and his research in cell wall deficient organisms, in tandem with that of the late Dr. Wyburn-Mason is relevant to all aspects of microbiology and much of clinical medicine.

Chelation therapy, controversially but widely used in cardiovascular disease, has implications for the prevention of cancer and degenerative disease by the removal of lead and other carcinogenic or toxic substances from the body. There is evidence that EDTA, the primary chelating agent, has anti-viral and antibacterial capabilities, and may well have a role in the treatment of AIDS.

18

DR. HANS SELYE

The late Dr. Hans Selye of the University of Montreal has probably influenced the thinking of more people than any other medical researcher. However, he has been more appreciated by informed laymen and workers in fields related to medicine than by the medical profession. The latter have acknowledged his eminence but largely ignored his lifetime research which concerned broad and general factors of health and disease, unconfined to any one system or specialty.

Dr. Selye's classic STRESS OF LIFE sets out the responses of the body to physical, emotional and chemical stimulae. He focused on the pituitary-adrenal axis as the pathway by which stimulae (stress) are translated into functional and organic changes within the body. The interactions of the pituitary, adrenals, thymus-lymphatics and gastro-intestinal function are the basis for the General Adaptation Syndrome (GAS) for which he is most noted. This, the sequence by which any disturbance or stress of the body is met by alarm, adaptation, and finally exhaustion, applies to its systems and tissues. Selye, working prior to the full development of cortisone, explained its actions, the pitfalls of its use and the basic metabolic relationships of the nervous and the endocrine systems. His insights, as pertinent today as when he formulated them, underlie almost all aspects

85

of AIDS but they have been ignored by researchers and workers in the area.

Dr. Selye was not a microbiologist but his work often concerned body responses to micro-organisms. These responses underlie body defenses against what he termed the pleuro-causal (from many causes) or idiopathic (of unknown etiology) diseases such as peptic ulcer, collagen disease, arthritis, cardiovascular disease and cancer. Selye considered these diseases to result from conditioning factors that are dependent upon a final precipitating stress for their clinical emergence. It is significant that pleomorphic organisms have been demonstrated in each of these conditions. In THE STRESS OF LIFE, Dr. Selye tells of producing acute arthritis in a rat by injecting it with exudative fluid from a cancer.

AIDS fits Selye's category of pleuro-causal disease; its conditioning factors are multiple and often sequential infections, augmented usually but not inevitably by the AIDS Virus. The resultant form of AIDS is determined by the adaptive capacity of the body defense systems and not just T-lymphocyte integrity. Disturbed adrenal defenses pertain to all aspects of AIDS; these are involved in kidney lesions (nephrosclerosis), blood vessel lesions (vasculitis), thrombo-hemorrhagic disorders (thrombocytopenia), lymphocyte depletions, and autoimmune phenomena. They also pertain to the widely assorted neurologic, endocrine and neoplastic elements of the disease.

AIDS Related Complex illustrates Selye's alarm stage of the Local Adaptation Syndrome. The body attempts to contain local lesions by pro-inflammatory hormones, predominantly the growth hormone (STS) of the pituitary and the mineral regulatory hormones of the adrenal cortex, of which Aldosterone is primary. These predominate over the anti-inflammatory hormones which are primarily pituitary (ACTH) and Cortisol (hydrocortisone) of the adrenal cortex; these latter also regulate carbohydrate, fat and protein metabolism.

Local inflammatory responses produced within lymph nodes are additive to what is now recognized as Acute Phase Responses. These latter are generalized body reactions from mediator substances known collectively as Interleukin I. Produced by blood monocytes and tissue phagocytes, they appear to protect against a wide variety of assaults to body tissues. They are credited with producing fever, night sweats, muscle aches from breakdown of protein into amino acids, increased sleep, and other nonspecific indications of illness. In the laboratory an elevated blood sedimentation rate, the presence of C-Reactive proteins, increased gamma globulins, and often in conditions other than AIDS, a moderately increased white blood cell count, are found. Interleukin II, which so strongly activates the immune system by its stimulating of T-lymphocytes, is also derived from Interleukin I. In AIDS Related Complex and Kaposi's sarcoma, the prominence of these manifestations indicates that the body is still capable of defense activities; the diminution of symptomatology and improvement in certain laboratory findings (such as the sedimentation rate) does not always indicate a real improvement in the patient.

If at this time, the body is heavily and generally stressed (as with multiple infections), the body shifts into the alarm stage of the General Adaptation Syndrome; there is a surge of pituitary ACTH which stimulates its target organ, the adrenal cortex. The latter floods the body with anti-inflammatory hormones; the thymus and lymphatic tissues shrink, the lymphocytes are reduced and the body loses much of its ability to react with inflammation. The adaptation stage can culminate in exhaustion and the stage is set for Opportunistic Infection.

Kaposi's sarcoma can be viewed as local manifestations of the General Adaptation Syndrome to the CMV or E.B. viruses and the Mycobacteria which have been reported in the lesions. The benign course of classic Kaposi's sarcoma probably relates to an age-related diminution or distortion of adrenal function, as well as poor tissue oxygenation. The Mycobacteria that have increasingly been noted in Kaposi lesions may have a causative role, or they may represent bacteria attracted to the area by the hemosiderin (iron) deposited there. Both Cytomegalovirus (CMV) and Mycobacteria have a predilection for the adrenals, and there they can diminish or destroy adrenal function.

Classic Kaposi lesions (and not Opportunistic Infections) are induced by the use of steroids and other immunosuppressive drugs; they often regress when the medications are discontinued and the patients show no evidence of cell mediated immunosuppression (low lymphocyte counts, T4T8 ratio reversals and depressed mitogen responses). This suggests a distortion of adrenal defenses rather than depressed cellular immunity or the altered complement-properdin systems that is present in Opportunistic Infection.

Kaposi's sarcoma, a central enigma of AIDS, is probably a connecting link between microbial pathogens and the formation of new tissue capable of evolving into malignancy.

Particularly pertinent is Selye's statement: "INFLAMMATION, ONE OF THE MOST STRIKING FEATURES OF LOCAL STRESS, IS ACCOMPANIED BY SELECTIVE TISSUE GROWTH AT THE SITE OF INJURY. Some of this is purely developmental (increase in size and number of cells) but some is re-developmental (transformation of connective tissue cells into other types). . . . Conditioning factors alter regional tissue responsiveness and permit selective reaction to hormones which are equally distributed to all parts of the body through the blood."

With or without Kaposi's sarcoma, Opportunistic Infection aligns with Selye's General Adaptation Syndrome stage of exhaustion. When nutritional, metabolic, enzymatic and endocrine reserves are over-stressed, damaged or inadequate, even chemotherapy, antibiotics and immunotherapy cannot avert the final stage. There is a depletion of adrenal substances, including adrenalin and nor-epinepherine balances, so that the parasympathetic autonomic nervous system predominates. As in Addison's Disease (in which the substance and function of the adrenals are destroyed), the body is unable to mount any appreciable inflammatory response to the multiple underlying infections; neither can it adequately produce the anti-inflammatory hormones which were marshalled in earlier stages. The terminal stage of Opportunistic Infection is identical to that of terminal cancer with a depletion of all aspects of defense and metabolic body function.

Aldosterone, the primary pro-inflammatory hormone, has received little attention in general medicine except for its mineral regulatory capacity but in the treatment of AIDS even this has been overlooked. Along with DOCA, a lesser pro-inflammatory hormone, it regulates sodium and potassium balances of the body. In adrenal insufficiency, the body pours out sodium from the kidneys and the bowels, inducing acidosis in many ARC and Opportunistic Infection patients. The often intractable diarrhea that can be such a distressing feature of this illness may well be attributed to this activity of the mineralcorticoids.

Adrenal depletion, and imbalances between the pro-inflammatory and anti-inflammatory hormones, are seldom recognized or treated. Probably the most pertinent and rational replacement therapy is Adrenal Cortical Extract, but this was eliminated from the market by the FDA in a much contested power play in 1978.* There are no readily available synthetic adrenal cortical hormones on the market having the pro-inflammatory capability that is so much needed in AIDS.

Every physician working with AIDS should be required to review adrenal physiology and read Selye's THE STRESS OF LIFE.

---

*page 156

19

PLEOMORPHIC (CELL WALL DEFICIENT) ORGANISMS

René Dubos, renowned microbiologist of the Rockefeller Institute, summarized the current state of microbiology: "We have inherited from the 19th century a very lopsided view of the problem of microbial diseases. We think of them as caused by a microbe that one catches from contaminated water or food, or from a sick person. This type of causation was indeed common in the past . . . (but) most microbial diseases today are caused by microbes which are ubiquitous in the community and indeed are present all the time in the body of normal individuals. Under usual conditions, these ubiquitous microbes do not cause any trouble. They persist . . . in a latent dormant form. But they can be brought into a state of activity and thus become the cause of a disease when some disturbance occurs which upsets the equilibrium."

Following the demonstration by Pasteur in the 1870s of microbes as a cause of disease, they were considered the cause of all disease, with the medical profession defending the doctrine as zealously as they had originally opposed it. The demonstration in the 1920s of vitamin deficiency states relaxed the emphasis on microbes, and a mid-century recognition that functional stress can lead to organic disease helped to move microbes from center stage as a primary cause of disease.

Today, an increasing incidence of chronic and degenerative diseases (including cancer, arthritis, multiple sclerosis, and collagen disease) is re-directing attention to a large amorphous group of organisms termed "pleomorphics" which can be found in these conditions and in AIDS. Pleomorphic organisms (those having two or more separate forms during a life cycle) have bedeviled microbiologists for over a century; they have variously been termed "Pleuro-Pneumonia Like Organisms (PPLOs)", "L" organisms (for the Lister Institute in England where Emmy Klieneberger-Nobel definitely established their bacteriologic classification), and descriptively as "Cell Wall Deficient Organisms" (CWDOs). Possessing complicated life cycles which alternate between bacterial and viral characteristics, they have aerobic (oxygen dependent) and anaerobic forms, poorly demonstrated by ordinary staining, culture or microscopy techniques, and they are able to alternate between forms with and without cell walls.

Mycoplasmas, although superficially identical to "L" organisms, are genetically incapable of forming cell walls so they are excluded from the category. They have, however, been accepted by medical science as valid pathogenic entities, capable of causing atypical pneumonia and much gynecologic disease. Many researchers have thought that Mycoplasmas might cause certain malignancies but the evidence points to pleomorphic organisms as more likely culprits.

Pleomorphic organisms are classical bacteria, fungi, and protozoa which adapt to physical and chemical agents, including antibiotics, enzymes, temperature, osmotic and pH (acid-alkaline) gradients of their environment so that they defensively lose their cell walls. Entering into complicated life cycles, interspersed cryptically and often intracellularly among tissues and organs of the body, they await proper conditions to regrow their walls and revert to their original and classifiable forms.

These organisms have been considered of minor clinical consequence, notable only as laboratory curiosities; they defy rigid classification and, blurring the distinctions between viruses and bacteria, they raise fundamental questions regarding genetic versus environmental transmission of characteristics. Pleomorphic organisms are demonstrable as the silent stage of a gamut of infections that include Tuberculosis, Syphilis, Leprosy, Rheumatic Fever, Undulant Fever, Typhoid and Candida. They have been repeatedly found in diseases of undetermined etiology: Arthritis, Cancer, Multiple Sclerosis, Sarcoid, Collagen Disease, Whipple's Disease and Crohn's Disease (both severe and poorly treatable chronic inflammatory diseases of the bowel) and Kaposi's Sarcoma.

Current recognition and interest in pleomorphic organisms is only a fresh chapter in a long and recurrent chronicle that began with Professor Antoine Beachamp (1816-1908) of the University of Toulouse, a contemporary of Pasteur. He advanced the Microzyme theory of disease that postulates for all bacteria a common ancestor that is scattered throughout nature and is present in all living organisms. He believed that the form and pathogenicity for any strain of bacteria is primarily determined by its environment, and that they participate in creating the conditions by which disease occurs, but are not themselves the primary cause of disease.

Beauchamp's concepts had little impact on conventional thought or bacteriologic doctrine in an era dominated by Pasteur but they provide the background for the exacting life work of Almquist (1852-1946), a Swedish bacteriologist and physician who provided a basis for almost all work in the field. Almquist had worked with Pasteur and also with Robert Koch, the German Nobel prize winner who discovered the Tubercule bacillus as the cause of Tuberculosis; Koch also noted but never investigated the pleomorphic forms of the Typhoid bacillus.

Pleomorphics have been a tolerated but not widely accepted field of microbiology. Almquist's research was followed by that of the Leyton's, Crofton and Klienberger-Nobel of Britain, von Brehmer of Germany, Gerlach of Austria, Tedeschi, Mori and Fonti.of Italy, Villequez and Roux of France and numerous other reputable researchers; Lohnis compiled an analysis of 1309 medical articles published between 1838 and 1919 dealing with observations and research in this area. In 1974 there was an international meeting devoted solely to these organisms, sponsored by the Societe Francaise de Microbiologie, at Montpelier, France.

In the United States, a bitter debate developed in the 1920s between the so-called "filtrationist" and "anti-filtrationist" schools of bacteriology. The filtrationists, represented by Dr. Kendall of Northwestern Medical School and Dr. Rosenow of California, held that many bacteria, depending on environmental circumstances, are capable of a complicated life cycle with spore-like forms that pass like viruses through bacterial filters. These organisms, growing within the laboratory or within the tissues of a host, await proper environmental conditions to revert to a bacteriologically recognizable and classifiable form. The anti-filtrationists, represented by Dr. Rivers of the Rockefeller Institute and Dr. Zinsser of Harvard, maintained that each species of bacteria is firmly and forever fixed within its own life cycle and cannot be affected by environmental conditions. All evidence to the contrary was held to be unscientific; the growth of organisms from filtrates was considered to be caused by poor laboratory techniques that allowed ordinary bacterial contamination of the culture media.

Despite the demonstration in California by the unorthodox genius, Royal Rife, that these organisms were clearly visible in human cancer specimens at a microscopic magnification of 30,000, the anti-filtrationists won out. The California Medical Society opposed Rife's unorthodox work and disciplined any physician suspected of dealing with or using his techniques or his instruments. Rife also demonstrated that by environmental and nutrient manipulation, he could convert one species of bacteria to another (ie: E. Coli to Typhoid) He postulated that there are approximately ten different classses of bacteria; within each class, the conversion of one type to another is a matter of environmental manipulation.

The past twenty five years have vindicated the filtrationists, but despite their increasing respectability, clinical bacteriologists have largely ignored pleomorphic organisms. Few laboratories are willing to perform the slow and meticulous work that is necessary to grow them. Dr. Louis Dienes of Boston quietly demonstrated the presence of these organisms and his precise and meticulous techniques enabled other bacteriologists to isolate them from diseased tissues; they have had trouble convincing the medical profession that these cause the illnesses with which they are found. Physicians have been reluctant to apply clinically the large volume of knowledge that is available regarding pleomorphs, and if they wish to engage in research are also reluctant to espouse controversial or unpopular areas of investigation.

From time to time, enterprising physicians have bridged the gap between laboratory and clinic. The late Dr. W.A. Altemeier of the University of Cincinnati first published evidence that pleomorphic organisms are a cause of both spontaneous and post-operative thrombophlebitis (infected blood clots in a vein) and in pulmonary emboli (blood clots which have broken off and lodged in the lung). Dr. Thomas McP. Brown, formerly of George Washington Medical School, has long demonstrated an involvement of cell wall defective organisms in Rheumatoid Arthritis; he has successfully treated them with antibiotics.

In 1976 Drs. Emil Wirostko and L.A. Johnson of Columbia University Medical Center inoculated mice with uveal fluid*

---

*page 179

(from the eyes) of patients with arthritis and collagen disease, and produced a spectrum of disease ranging from arthritis to hepatitis, with almost all the mice dead by eight months. Dr. G.J. Domingue of Tulane Medical School has extensively demonstrated that much kidney disease is associated with inapparent infections of cell wall deficient organisms. It is tempting to consider that many kidney transplants and renal dialyses might be preventable by proper diagnosis and treatment of underlying pleomorphic infections.

The major authorities in the pleomorphic field have been Guze of Stanford, Haflick of U. of California, Mattman of Wayne State University and Domingue of Tulane; each of them has edited definitive surveys of the field in 1967, 1969, 1974 and 1982 respectively.

The thread that ties diverse illnesses and pleomorphic organisms together is that of stressed body defenses. When the reticuloendothelial system is compromised by psychologic, physiologic or chemical stress, growth restraints are released from normally innocuous microbes and they transform into cell wall deficient variants incorporated within the body tissues and organs for which the different organisms appear to have a specific affinity. It is thought their genetic material can be introduced into the cell and expressed on the cell membrane, thereby provoking an attack from either humoral or cellular components of the immune system. The resultant autoimmune disease can include Hemolytic Anemia, thyroid, renal or vascular disease (including Vasculitis and Lupus Erythematosis) or neuromuscular conditions, such as Multiple Sclerosis. Cox has demonstrated that anemia associated with red blood inclusions, such as the malarial parasite, is an immune response against the red blood cell itself; this mechanism could relate to the anemias of cancer, arthritis and other conditions in which micro-organisms can be found in the red blood cells.

The beneficial results obtained in many of these conditions

by non-specific bacterial vaccines are attributed to the stimulation of the reticuloendothelial system. Beneficial results obtained from immuno-modulating compounds (which are generally effective against parasites, and often belong to the Imidazole family) might be from a direct chemical attack upon an organism unprotected by a cell wall (eg: the amoebae of Dr. Wyburn-Mason).*

The presence of pleomorphic organisms in AIDS has been an unnoted factor in its wide systemic and organ involvements. These microbes (bacterial, viral, fungal and protozoal), shaped by wide disturbances of the internal environment, are difficult to separate into individual components. The conversion of normal intestinal microbes into pathogenic "L" forms by altered nutritional status, antibiotics and parasites undoubtedly has a role in this aspect of AIDS.

In 1911, Peyton Rous of the Rockefeller Institute demonstrated that sarcoma, a widespread malignancy in chickens, could be produced by inoculating healthy fowls with an extract of diseased tissue, which, because of its filterability was presumed to be a virus. As recognition for his achievement, he was awarded the Nobel Prize in 1926. Rous's work was confirmed in Britain by the Leytons and by Crofton; the latter, a longtime prolific worker with pleomorphic organisms, was prominent for his use of autogenous vaccines (made from organisms cultured from the patient) in the treatment of infections as well as cancer.

As early as 1890, William Russell, a Scottish Pathologist had reported on widely variagated microbes present in all cancer tissue. The exact origin and composition of the "Russell bodies" he observed has never been definitively determined but recurrently they are implicated as pleomorphic organisms. James Young, a Scottish obstetrician, also reported on the life cycles of "parasites" which he observed in cancer tissue. Similar work

---

*Chapter 21

was later done in California by Drs. Sturdivant and Stearn, and in Chicago by Dr. John Nuzum.

Dr. George Mazet of France reported on "acid-fast" bacteria in Hodgkins disease and leukemia in the 1940's but it was the German von Brehmer's 1930's demonstration of the life cycle of pleomorphic organisms (which he termed "Syphonospora Polymorpha") that is the reference point for all subsequent (and current) work within the field.

In the United States, the clinically directed pleomorphic-cancer tradition began with Dr. T.J. Glover, whose serum, obtained from organisms grown from cancer tissue, is now generally considered to have been originated by Glover's assistant, Thomas Deaken. They are credited with having cultured organisms from over 3,000 cancer patients and with inducing verified cancer remissions with their serum in an appreciable number of them. Glover's work was taken up by Dr. M.J. Scott, a surgeon who devoted his life to a fruitless attempt at gaining official validation and recognition of the therapy.

The primary inheritor of the pleomorphic cancer tradition today is Dr. Virginia Livingston-Wheeler of California. In 1947 she demonstrated the presence of acid fast Mycobacteria in a patient with Scleroderma (a collagen disease of the skin) and reported its successful treatment with an antibiotic. The organism, injected into mice, produced scleroderma-like lesions, as well as cancer, in a number of them, thereby launching Dr. Livingston-Wheeler into her untiring career in cancer research. In 1948 she published the first of her many reports on the presence of these organisms in cancer. She and Dr. Eleanor Alexander Jackson placed the organism within the order Actinomycetales and named it "progenitor Cryptocides" (hidden, ancestral killer). Their work in the culture of pleomorphic organisms from all types of cancer and the production of cancer in animals from these organisms, has been corroborated and paralleled by Drs. William and Irene Diller and by Dr. Florence Seibert. In the

1930s, Dr. George Clark of the Department of Public Health in Washington, spent eight years reproducing and validating Glover's work in the production of animal tumors from cultures derived from cancer, but his research was not presented in public until 1953 at the Sixth International Congress of Microbiology in Rome.

Dr. Eleanor Alexander Jackson has also demonstrated an "L" phase in the life cycle of the Tuberculosis bacillus and of Leprosy. She also has demonstrated that the Rous virus is not a virus but the viral-like phase of a pleomorphic organism, as is the material present in the Bittner mouse milk, which transmits breast cancer from mother to daughter mouse of that strain.

While Drs. Jackson, Diller and Seibert have worked within the protection and respectability of the laboratory, Dr. Livingston-Wheeler has also worked in the clinic. She has used her Cryptocides vaccine and a health-oriented approach to a wide range of degenerative disease, including cancer. Restoration of body defenses is the primary object of therapy, and any improvement in underlying disease is secondary. The Livingston-Wheeler regime includes diet, stock bacterial vaccines (including BCG, a live, weakened strain of the Tuberculosis bacillus), enzymes, her Cryptocides vaccine cultured from the patient, vitamin-mineral combinations, and nutritional combinations to provide the system with Abscissic acid. Dr. Livingston, perceiving that the latter, (a plant constituent related to Vitamin A but commercially unavailable, might be applicable as an adjunct in cancer therapy, originated a method of producing it by nutritional combinations in her cancer diet.

Prominent among Dr. Livingston-Wheeler's contributions is her demonstration that pleomorphic organisms found in spermatozoa, like those in cancer tissue, are capable of producing choriogonadatrophin (CG), a mammalian hormone that protects its producer-carriers from destruction by body defenses. Her work, confirmed by Drs. Hernan Acevedo of the University of

Pittsburg and Louis Affronti of George Washington University, has opened a fresh field of cancer research in which neutralization of CG may prove a therapeutic tool against cancer.

That abscissic acid may be a potent anti-CG material justifies its consideration in cancer regimes. A small jig saw piece in the cancer puzzle is Sialic Acid (a constituent of CG) whose lipid-bound form, a marker for the presence of cancer activity, pregnancy and AIDS, is elevated in the former and depressed in the latter two conditions). It has been suggested that the highly negative ionic charge of Sialic Acid within the CG repels the negatively charged lymphocytes and macrophages of the immune system, thereby protecting sperm, fetal tissue and cancer cells from immunologic attack.

Unexplained thrombophlebitis and embolic episodes, are often an early manifestation of cancer and pleomorphic organisms can be found in both conditions. The late Dr. Guy Owens, surgeon of Amarillo, Texas, and his laboratory assistant, Paul Miranda, noting the presence of pleomorphic organisms in blood smears of cancer patients, kept records of their findings. Twenty three out of twenty five patients with organisms in their blood but no clinical evidence of cancer, developed cancer over a twenty year period of time.*

In 1975, the Department of Microbiology of Sloan Kettering Institute undertook to prove or disprove the existence of pleomorphic organisms in blood taken from cancer patients. When organisms were grown from all the blood cultures, the growths were ascribed to outside contamination and the project discarded as flawed.

Medical Establishment acceptance of the relevance and validity of pleomorphic organisms will pose countless problems and challenges for the medical profession, far beyond their possible role in AIDS.

---

*page 101

Cell Wall-Deficient Bacteria
Basic Principles and Clinical Significance

Gerald J. Domingue, *Editor*

Tulane University School of Medicine
New Orleans, Louisiana

1982

ADDISON-WESLEY PUBLISHING COMPANY
Advanced Book Program/World Science Division
Reading, Massachusetts

London   Amsterdam   Don Mills, Ontario   Sydney   Tokyo

CONTRIBUTORS

CAROLYN L. BARTH. Department of Pathology. Henry Ford Hospital. Detroit, Michigan

BLAINE L. BEAMAN. Department of Medical Microbiology. University of California School of Medicine. Davis, California

ALAN R CANTWELL, JR. Department of Dermatology. Southern California Permanente Medical Group. Los Angeles, California

GERALD J DOMINGUE. Department of Urology and Department of Microbiology and Immunology Tulane University School of Medicine. New Orleans, Louisiana

RICHARD W GiLPIN. Department of Microbiology. The Medical College of Pennsylvania and Hospital. Philadelphia, Pennsylvania

JAMES C. GRAY. Department of Biological Sciences. Wayne State University. Detroit, Michigan

PAUL M. HEIDGER, JR. Department of Anatomy. University of Iowa School of Medicine. Iowa City, Iowa

PHILIP C. HESSBURG. Detroit Institute of Ophthalmology. Grosse Pointe. Michigan

MEHNGA S. JUDGE. College of Medicine. Wayne State University. Detroit, Michigan

GYTA KAGAN. Gamaleya Institue of Epidemiology and Microbiology. Academy of Medical Sciences, Moscow. Russia

WILLIAM J LARSEN. Department of Anatomy. University of Cincinnati School of Medicine. Cincinnati. Ohio

JOHN W LAWSON Department of Microbiology. Clemson University. Clemson. South Carolina

RAYMOND J LYNN Department of Microbiology The University of South Dakota School of Medicine. Vermillion. South Dakota

LIDA H MATTMAN. Department of Biological Sciences. Wayne State University. Detroit, Michigan

PAUL D MITCHELL. Section of Clinical Microbiology. Marshfield Clinic, St. Joseph's Hospital. Marshfield. Wisconsin

EDWARD A MOSCOVIC. Medizinische Hochschule Hannover. Hannover, West Germany, and Medizinische Hochschule Hannover. Hannover. West Germany

KEVIN PARENT. Section of Gastroenterology. Marshfield Clinic, St. Joseph's Hospital. Marshfield. Wisconsin

SUZANNE K. PATTERSON. Merck. Sharp and Dohme Research Laboratories. West Point. Pennsylvania

JANINE SCHMITT SLOMSKA. Institut National de la Santé et de la Recherche Médicale U 65. Universite de Montpellier I. Faculte de Médecine. Nimes. France

PAUL F. SMITH. Department of Microbiology. The University of South Dakota School of Medicine. Vermilion. South Dakota

T. WOODIE SMITH JR. Department of Biological Sciences. Gulf Coast Community College. Panama City. Florida

PATRICK D. WALKER Department of Pathology. Tulane University School of Medicine. New Orleans Louisiana

HANNAH B WOODY. Department of Pediatrics. Tulane University School of Medicine. New Orleans, Louisiana

DAVID WRAY. Laboratory of Oral Medicine. National Institute of Dental Research National Institute of Health, Bethesda. Maryland

C-O-P-Y

Amarillo, Tex.
1-18-1979

Dear Dr. Brown:

Thank you for your kind and interesting letter and the enclosures.
I am working constantly as best I can on my version of a causative
bacteria in malignancy. This started in 1945 when Paul Miranda, a
lab technician observed motile cocci-like organisms in a red blood
cell while he was looking for Rocky Mountain Spotted Fever. Mr Miranda
came to work with me and we both began to wonder about his finding,
especially when we learned from the patient that he had cancer.

From this, we started to look into all the malignancy cases we
could find and struggled to make this a diagnostic tool. We were
never able to find above 40% of malignancies showing clearly a parasitic
infection of the red cells but we became more and more aware of the
magnitude of the numbers of this organism in the circulating blood,
especially in terminal cases. We began to look for the organism in
every blood count we made and to our surprise we began to pick up a
few cases with the bacteria in sufficient numbers to be identified
during a blood count. No cases of parasitic red cell infestation
were found in these cases even when our special stain was used in looking
for this condition. We selected 25 cases from my practice where the
organism was repeatedly found during blood counts. They were run of
the mill office cases, being male, female, old and young but apparently
in averagely good health. Over a twenty year period, twenty three of
these people came down with malignancy of one kind or another....proven
by surgery and proper pathologic examination. Two cases were lost from
our records although one was known to have died from an obscure abdom-
inal condition. This is of course an insignificant number of cases
but it was enough to make an impact on our thinking about the significance of the organism we were working with.

I have visited with Dr. Eleanor Jackson and Dr. Virginia Livingston
and both were wonderful and anxious to be of any help to me that they
could be. There is no doubt that their Cryptocides and our organism
is the same. Dr. Livingstone is frank in giving credit to the many
people in the past who have observed and worked with the organism
but she deserves credit for doing more constructive work with it than
anyone else. Her use of the dark field is most important; since using
this I have studied over 100 bloods with the dark field and am forced
to believe that every individual carries this unusual organism around
with him from birth to death.

I am shocked at the number of acid fast organisms found on smearing
formalin preserved malignant tissues. I do not understand why more
bacteriological investigative work in malignancy is not done. This
organism can be identified in many tissues since it circulates freely
in the blood stream. I know white blood cells pick them up .but I
lack the necessary processes to identify them properly in white cells..

.... sincerely:

Guy Owens MD F.A.C.S.

20

GASTON NAESSENS

A resolution for the role of pleomorphic organisms in health and disease resides in the Canadian microscope of Gaston Naessens. Using ultraviolet and lasar beam technology, it magnifies up to 30,000 and duplicates many of the findings of the controversial Rife microscope of the 1940s. Unlike electron microscopy, which works only with the dried and fixed remains of what is studied, the Naessens "Somatoscope" demonstrates living organisms with unparalleled clarity, and makes possible time lapse studies of evolving organisms.

The Naessens story began in 1963 when Gaston Naessens, a previously obscure French biologist, blazed into public attention by providing physicians with an apparently successful cancer therapy. Prosecuted and fined in 1956 for practicing medicine without a license, he had thereafter refrained from treating patients but had made his products available to physicians in France and Switzerland.

"L'Affair Naessens" erupted when stories appeared in the public media of the success of his anti-cancer serum Anablast in the treatment of childhood leukemia, that at the time was medically untreatable. In an unprecedented carnival of widely reported frenzy, parents with sick children besieged Corsica where Naessens was living. As Naessens would not treat the children himself, and few physicians were willing to become embroiled in such a controversial matter, there were demonstrations and protests to the government to investigate and make available for public use this apparently successful cancer therapy. The situation closely paralleled the Krebiozin trials of the same era in the United States. Both were issues of medical authority challenged by apparently successful treatments that followed neither orthodox theory nor conventional practices. Naessens's case was additionally serious in that he was not an MD.

The investigation, conducted and reported under the direction of the French Ministry of Health, was ferocious and merciless. In a travesty of impartial investigation, all testimony or evidence of patient improvement was thrown out and the final expert opinion against Naessens was so overwhelming that he was again brought to trial for practicing medicine and pharmacy without a licence. His conviction was accompanied by court costs and the maximum fine allowed by the law. In its judgement, the court regretted that a heavier penalty could not have been imposed. That was the end of L'Affair Naessens.

In retrospect, the inability of French medical authorities to investigate impartially or to recognize the possibility that Anablast might be effective is that it was a serum derived from pleomorphic organisms. These were isolated independently by Naessens, but paralleled closely Glover's serum, the vaccine of Crofton, of Krebiozin, and currently, the Cryptocides vaccine of Livingston, all of which have been inexplicable to establishment authories. Also, Naessens was unsophisticated, stubborn and naive in dealing with medical and court authorities and did little to help his cause. One report on the trial comments that "He evinces neither humility nor submission to criticism, which are the best qualities of a scientist."

After the investigation and trials, Naessens fled to Canada where he has worked in his privately supported laboratory on the relevance of these organisms to all areas of biology. He has gained stature among an increasing number of scientists who, unperturbed by his unorthodoxy, have investigated his work.

Naessen's work, based on his microscope, delivers a new basis for the entire field of biology far beyond demonstrating the presence of cell wall deficient organisms in all areas of disease. It demonstrates that there is an ecologic framework within the body by which micro-organisms are moulded and within which is the impetus for mammalian cell division. It is squarely in the tradition of Beauchamp, who postulated a common progenitor for all bacteria, and of Rife, who demonstrated the existence of interchangeable types of bacteria, whose forms are determined by environmental conditions. It delivers a fresh approach for the control and treatment of cancer and of much degenerative disease.

THE SOMATID (by Gaston Naessens)

The standard microscope permits a maximal enlargement to 1800X with a maximal resolution (index of clarity) of 0.1 micron. The electron microscope can achieve an enlargement into the millions with a resolution of 30 to 50 angstroms but the object of study must be dried and fixed so that only its skeletal outlines can be seen.

Using a combination of Laser and ultraviolet technology, we have developed an instrument which we call the "Somatoscope" that permits the observation of living organisms up to a magnification of 30,000 with a resolution of 150 angstroms. Because of the infinite time and intricacies of working at the higher magnifications, most of our work has been done at the lower ranges.

With this instrument, we have observed in all biologic liquids, and particularly in the blood, an elementary particle endowed with movement and possessing a variable life cycle of many forms. We have called this particle a "somatid" and in the proper media, it can be isolated and cultured. Its dimensions vary from a few angstroms to 0.1 of a micron and it is present in the blood of all individuals. It is the diversity of forms emerging in many disease states that distinguishes their possessors from healthy individuals.

We postulate and have evidence that the normal life cycle of this organism consists of somatids, spores and double spores and that these produce a hormone-like substance (which we have termed "trefons", after the usage of Alexis Carrel, that initiate cell division within the body. In healthy individuals, the somatid cycle is regulated and controlled by blood inhibitors (usually certain trace minerals and organic substances).

If, due to stress or other biologic disturbances, these inhibitors within the blood are diminished, the relatively simple cycle of somatids, spores and double spores is diverted into another and more elaborate cycle; one then sees within the tissues, and particularly within the blood, the diverse forms of bacteria known as Syphonospora Polymorpha that were so well demonstrated by the German scientist von Brehmer in the 1930s. Within this group can be placed the wide range of mutable organisms that have been variously described as "Pleomorphic Organisms," "L" forms, or "Cell Wall Deficient Organisms".

Little is known of bacterial evolution; there is no really adequately comprehensive classification for many microbial forms but it appears that the infinite variations of pleomorphic bacteria that are present in many disease states can be aligned within the expanded somatid cycle. They can be aerobic, anaerobic, motile or non-motile, with varying staining capacity (especially for Gram and acid-fast stains). The accompanying diagram* demonstrate their forms which can range from coccal (ie: Streptococcus and Staphylococcus) to baccillary (from the

---

*page 118

rod like forms of Mycobacteria to the curves of spirochetes). The pathogenically prominent Mycobacteria evolve and burst (Eclatment), releasing yeast-like "levurids" at a level which can be termed "fungal" although this term applies more to the appearance than the physical characteristics of the organisms. The "levurids" evolve through "ascospores" to "asci" which are indistinguishable by ordinary laboratory means from small lymphocytes. Forming cytoplasm, the "asci" in an adequately nutritious environment develop as "thalli" whose walls burst and liberate an enormous quantity of new somatids that initiate another complete cycle. The fibrous thallus, emptied of its cytoplasm and contents, is often observed on stained smears and catalogued and dismissed as being an artifact. (Except to call them "fibrin formations", no one has ever explained the wide prevalence of these "artifacts" in carefully prepared and usually sterile slides!!)

In our laboratory we can show that derivatives of the somatid cycle, and other substances that react with these organisms, are capable of effects that pertain to many current problems and challenges of medicine. They are relevant to cancer, organ transplantation and many aspects of degenerative diseases.

(See Illustrations Starting on Page 118)

21

DR. ROGER WYBURN-MASON

The late Dr. Roger Wyburn-Mason of Britain is high on any list of brilliant but controversial physicians. Despite impressive academic and professional credentials, with a long and solid medical background in research and clinic, his major medical contribution is still controversial. However, an increasing number of physicians are using his methods and investigating his laboratory work.

In 1975, while participating in a symposium on fungal disease, he reported a series of rheumatoid arthritis patients whom he had successfully treated with Chlortrimazole, a broad spectrum anti-fungal and anti-parasitic medication. This was immediately reported by the news media and clamor arose around the world as patients besieged their physicians for this new medical treatment.

Dr. Wyburn-Mason postulated that Entamoeba Limax, a species of protozoa (one celled organisms belonging to the animal kingdom) found extensively throughout nature, and present in almost all living creatures, can cause a wide spectrum of degenerative disease, including arthritis, cancer and collagen disease. He demonstrated the presence of amoeba by special collecting and staining techniques, and he reported impressive therapeutic results by using a wide assortment of anti-fungal and anti-parasitic medications.

The Medical Establishment loftily denied the validity of Dr. Wyburn-Mason's theory or his results and deplored his failure to use double blind studies or to obtain official recognition and approval before publicly announcing his results. Attention was directed toward Dr. Wyburn-Mason's less attractive personality traits and actions but the major objection to his work was that it did not fit conventional patterns of thought or practice. Almost all rheumatologists and medical organizations deplored his work, but no one officially investigated or evaluated the patients for whom treatment had been successful.

Chloroquin (Aralen), a standard treatment for malaria and other protooan infections, has long been known to be effective in rheumatoid arthritis although its side effects (primarily visual damage), have discouraged its wide use for this purpose. The majority of the anti-fungal and anti-protozoal medications used and advocated by Dr. Wyburn-Mason have been under investigation and use as potent modulators of the immune system. These are also allied to the use of Flagyl; in Britain, this is used as a potent antibiotic against anaerobic bacteria (those that thrive in a low oxygen environment). In the United States, its primary use is against Trichomonas, a vaginal infection from a low-grade, widely prevalent protozoa.

Despite the unorthodoxy of Dr. Wyburn-Mason's therapies, an increasing number of physicians have tried them and found them effective. In the United States, the Rheumatoid Disease Foundation has been established to coordinate and dispense information regarding the therapy, with the primary goal of achieving a proper evaluation and recognition of its medical value. The first national meeting of physicians using this approach was held in Birmingham Alabama in July 1985.

It appears that Entamoeba Limax, as a cell wall deficient

protozoa, normally present in the body and demonstrable in a wide spectrum of disease, aligns in almost all essentials with bacterial cell-wall deficient organisms. It is likely that the Naessens microscope, by re-arranging the field of microbiology, may bring the associated but neglected field of clinical protozoology into focus.

THE
RHEUMATOID DISEASE FOUNDATION

RT. 4, BOX 137, FRANKLIN, TN 37064 / (615) 646-1030

PERRY A. CHAPDELAINE, SR.
Executive Director-Secretary

March 14, 1985

Dear **Dr. Brown:**

I am enclosing Professor Roger Wyburn-Mason's latest publication (*A Precis' and Addendum*), which should give you the basis for some of his findings. He announced his work at the IXth International Conference of Chemotherapy (London 1975). I understand he received a standing ovation, but no one followed up on his work.

In addition to his medical degree, Roger Wyburn-Mason had a Ph.D. in protozoology. In 1958 Henry Kimpton published his book *The Reticulo-Endothelial System in Growth and Tumor Formation* and in 1964 Charles C. Thomas published *A New Protozoon — Its Relation to Malignant and Other Diseases*. It is hardly likely that he would confuse macrophages with *Acanthamoeba* or *Naegleria*, the two indicted limax amoeba.

Regarding cancer: Professor Roger Wyburn-Mason never claimed that amoebae directly caused all cancers. He stated that the limax amoeba set up the precursor conditions that lead to cancer — perhaps as much as 20%; and he suggested that killing the limax amoeba with antiamoebics could very well be a cancer preventive.

We are currently financing double-blind studies on clotrimazole at Bowman Gray School of Medicine, and will soon be funding three universities in duplicating Dr. Wyburn-Mason's reports on isolating out the limax amoebae and culturing it to satisfy Koch's postulate. We need funding to test out (double-blind), in addition, metronidazole, allopurinol, furazolidone, rifampicin, iodoquinol, PABA, tinidazole — all of which seem effective to different genus, species, strains, as per attached (*in vitro*) chemosensitivity tests, and in clinical practice (*in vivo*).

We surely concur with your conclusions — and note that the limax amoeba was found to carry the Legionaire's virus, according to the references attached.

We are not ourselves sure that either *Acanthamoeba* or *Naegleria* is involved, and it may or may not be *Entamoeba limax* — or perhaps one of the mycoplasmic amoebae. But surely our studies in protozoology will satisfy requirements of science when completed.

If I can help further, please advise.

Cordially,

Perry A. Chapdelaine, Sr.

THE RHEUMATOID DISEASE FOUNDATION IS A PROJECT OF
THE ROGER WYBURN-MASON & JACK M. BLOUNT FOUNDATION
FOR THE ERADICATION OF RHEUMATOID DISEASE

TAX EXEMPTION APPROVED BY THE UNITED STATES INTERNAL REVENUE SERVICE
CHARTERED STATE OF TENNESSEE / SOLICITATION PERMIT APPROVED

22

Emanuel Revici, MD

D r. Emanuel Revici, Roumanian born physician and scientist who arrived in New York shortly after World War II, has probably aroused more emotional reaction among segments of the Medical Establishment than any other medical researcher and clinician. His research accomplishments are awesome as are the implications of his clinical work. He is comparatively unknown to the general public in this country but not in Europe. He was the first physician to recognize the role of selenium in the prevention and treatment of cancer, having delivered a paper on it in the 1960s. His anti-bleeding agent "Hemostypticum Revici" has long been a standard drug in Europe. Dr. Revici's patients have ranged from all varieties of celebrities to Catholic bishops and addicts (drug, alcohol and tobacco).

His voluminous and wide ranging work at his Institute of Applied Biology has never been accepted by orthodox research publications but is presented in his 1961 book "Research in Physiopathology as Basis of Guided Chemotherapy". (D. Van Nostrand Company Ltd.) It is the distillation of the work of a unique medical genius, centering around the concept of all phases of biology as opposing forces, comparable to the Yin-Yang concepts of the Orient.

In the 1970s, Dr. Revici directed a successful narcotics treatment center. Despite extensive publicity, including a Congressional hearing, and the evidence from two thousand successfully treated addicts, their physicians and agency representatives, Dr. Revici's program was discontinued. This was attributed to political pressures from the Medical Establishment.

The products used in the Revici therapy of alcoholism, narcotics addiction and tobacco habituation were extensively investigated and taken up for commercial development by several large companies but the projects were eventually discontinued. Presumably, this was because of the high cost, long time involvement, and slight chance of satisfying the FDA requirements for any new drug.

Dr. Revici's methods and materials are applicable to AIDS research and therapy; he reports encouraging results in AIDS Related Complex, Kaposi's sarcoma and Opportunistic Infection. To state an extreme simplification of his methods, he restores immunocompetency by reestablishing the disturbed sterols and fatty acid balances of the body; this is then supplemented by his anti-viral agents to clear the underlying viral infections.

Dr. Revici characterizes the opposing forces underlying all aspects of life and operating through all phases of body organization, as anabolic or catabolic. He postulates all aspects of body organization as beginning with sub-atomic particles and progressing to include chromosomes, nuclei, cells, tissues and organs. Each of these organizational levels emerges from the preceding one by incorporating aspects of its environment as an essential but secondary part. Compatible to this concept, Dr. Revici considers that all life started in mud, with animal life evolving from the sea and incorporating the sodium chloride there in its extracellular fluid; potassium, which occupies the same role in plants as sodium in the animal kingdom, is evidence that plants continued their evolution from within the mud (earth) and not, as generally believed, from the sea.

Dr. Revici's unifying characterization of physiology focuses on cell integrity and function as dependant on membrane equilibrium between fatty acids and sterols. He has demonstrated that the effectiveness of any therapeutic agent depends largely on its anabolic or catabolic activity correcting the imbalances's specific within each organizational level; elements from the periodic table align horizontally to each level of body organization with the heavier molecular weights progressively effective at the lower levels.

Dr. Revici's methods are not easily understood so few other physicians have used them. As they involve a combination of chemical and biologic products, produced by Dr. Revici, it is unlikely they will ever be available for use in this country.

23

THE RELEVANCE OF CHELATION

Lead, the legacy of the auto age, is the prototype for the effects of industrial pollution on health, working through the enzyme systems to devastate the metabolism of the body. Its effects are most evident on the nervous system; it stunts the mental and physical development of children, produces mental aberration and behavioral problems in the adult, and has increasingly been implicated in cancer formation.

In the 1940s it was found that EDTA (the di-sodium salt of Ethylene-diamine-tetra-acetic acid), intravenously administered to victims of lead poisoning, binds (chelates) the lead so it can then be excreted through the kidneys. During the course of therapy, it was found that X-ray evidence of arteriosclerotic deposits in the aorta and the arteries of the patients diminished; circulation in the extremities and vital organs appeared to be improved and many patients reported relief of various clinical symptoms, including intractable anginal pain. These serendipitous results were attributed to EDTA's affinity for other minerals, including calcium, which bind arteriosclerotic plaques to blood vessel walls.

Lead poisoning is the only officially approved indication for chelation therapy but as a non-surgical therapy for arteriosclerosis and cardiovascular disease it has gained increasing acceptance among health oriented physicians and the public. It has been strongly opposed by orthodox medicine although it was initially developed in an academic framework, with reports published in proper journals. As its use became widespread, so did official opposition; there have been no further presentations of the procedure in the meetings or the publications of the Medical Establishment except to condemn it.

Ostensibly, the basis for opposition to chelation is that it does not meet acceptable standards of investigation with double-blind studies (the Office of Technology in 1978 reported that only 10 to 20 percent of currently used medical procedures have been proven in controlled trials). A more likely explanation for widespread opposition to chelation therapy is that it competes with many aspects of conventional cardiology and eliminates much vascular surgery. It is thereby a threat to the financial interests of many physicians and the hospitals with which they are affiliated.

The toxic effect of lead on the macrophage system of the body contributes to malfunction of the immune system. There is a possibility that despite the controversy over its efficacy, chelation therapy may play a role in cancer prevention, as adjunctive therapy in AIDS, and across many areas of degenerative disease.

Probably the most advanced work in the development of atheroma (the predominantly cholesterol-calcium deposits that are the central factor of arteriosclerosis) and its treatment by chelation therapy is being done by Dr. A. Zeichmeister of the University of Bruno in Czechoslovakia. He has demonstrated the integration of trace minerals in cell function and the means of their therapeutic manipulations by chelation. Parenthetically, his demonstration of the damaging role of the Vitamin D. analogues on endothelium (the lining cells of blood vessels) aligns with the unnoted work of Dr. Hans Selye and of Dr. Mildred Seeley and the warnings of many nutritionists of this health hazard to the population.

Removing lead, cadmium, mercury, and other heavy metals from the body improves or corrects the enzyme systems poisoned by them; consequently all aspects of defense and metabolic functions of the body are enhanced.

That lead inactivates macrophages may relate to evidence that chelation therapy has a bearing on the prevention of cancer (and by implication on its treatment) as well as on other illnesses connected with lead toxicity. Dr. Walter Blumer of Switzerland, investigating the high cancer mortality among patients living along a highway suffused with lead from automotive traffic, has reported that chelated patients developed only one tenth the cancer as untreated controls living in the same locality. Dr. Blumer has also reported on the wide variety of neurologic and psychiatric illnesses he has improved or cured by chelation therapy.

Buried among the voluminous papers that have been published on chelation therapy, are two directly bearing on AIDS: Wunderlich in the Archives of Virology '82, 73 (21) pp171-83 reports on "The Disintegration of Retroviruses by Chelating Agents". An article in the 14 July 1984 issue of Lancet 14 (2) pp8394-99, refers to the efficacy of EDTA when used with previously ineffective antibiotics against Proteus pneumonia, a particularly intractable disease. There are also Russian references to the use of EDTA in the treatment of burn lesion infections, and also its modification of Staphylococcal sensitivity to pencillin.

Affecting viral and bacterial replication by mineral manipulations is a new concept, but it is consistent with much nutritional research dealing with trace minerals and their role in health and disease. It also emphasizes that mineral imbalances from the diarrheas of the Gay Bowel Syndrome may be pertinent in the decreased body defenses that are the background for AIDS. There are unofficial reports that patients whose blood on dark field examination shows many pleomorphic organisms will, immediately after chelation, be clear of them.

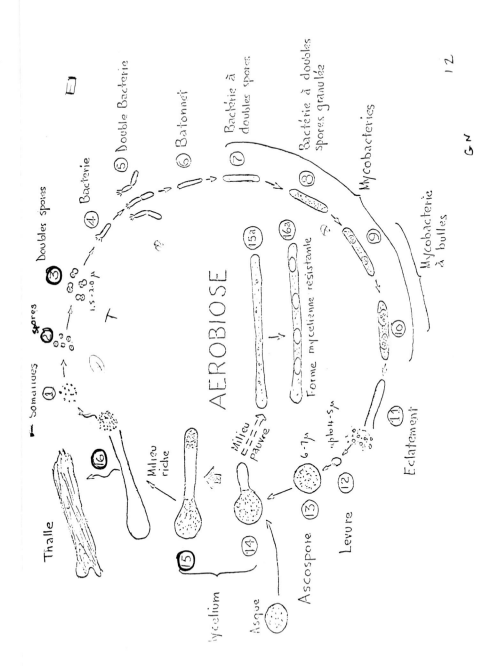

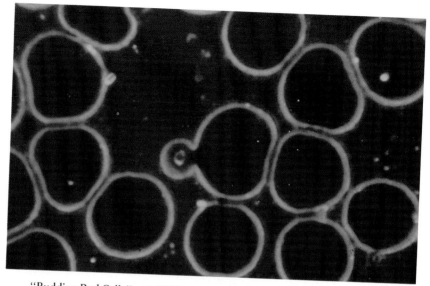

"Budding Red Cells" at 3,000X magnification

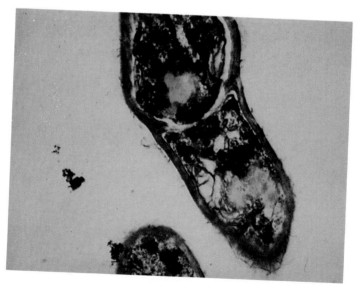

Asque developing Mycelium 30,000X magnification

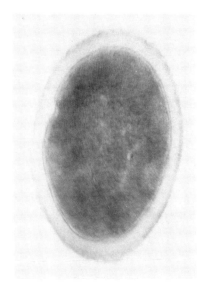

SPORE 30,000X MAGNIFICATION

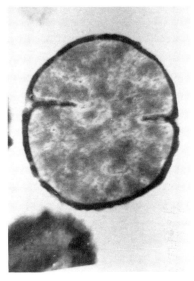

DIVIDING SPORE 20,000X

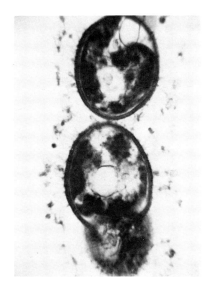

ASCOSPORES

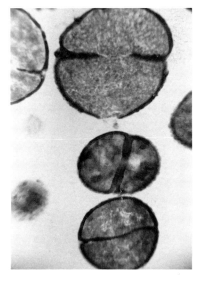

DOUBLE SPORES

Boguslaw Lipinski
37 Beaumont ...
Newton, MA 02..
(617) 527 1395

TO WHOM IT MAY CONCERN

In November 1979 I visited Mr.Gaston Naessens in his residence at Rock Forest in Canada. The purpose of my visit was to evaluate his research pertaining to the novel method of treatment of cancer. Mr Naessens has demonstrated for me his microscope and I have used my own blood sample to observe **somatides** floating freeley in plasma amongst the red cells. I have also seen a film showing **somatides** at various stages of proliferation in the blood of cancer patients.

In addition, my attention was attracted to an invention by Mr.Naessens which consists in a relatively simple formula and which, when injected into a limb of an animal, causes a painless and uncomplicated separation within 48 to 72 hours. I took back to Boston some of this solution and tested it in my laboratory (Department of Research, St.Elizabeth's Hospital of Boston) on one rat. To my surprise its leg separated within 24 hours leaving practically no wound! This experiment and my observation of Mr.Naessens work convinced me that he is a genuine scientists, despite the fact that he has no formal degrees.

In conclusion, I believe that Mr.Naessens work should be given a proper attention in order to fully explore the potential value of his research for the benefit of humanity. It might turn out that the cure for cancer is already available. Mr Gaston Naessens work may prove once more that it is not money but an inspiration and right intentions that bring progress to Science.

Boston, July 12, 1985   Boguslaw Lipinski, Ph.D.,D.Sc.

appendix "j"

24

THE CHALLENGE FROM THE WINGS

The AIDS virus is unofficially considered to affect macrophages, whose diminished production of Interleukin I (also known as acute phase substances), by lowering the level of Interleukin II, can interfere with T-lymphocyte function. The AIDS virus likewise affects granulocytes (polymorphonuclear white cells) that as part of the phagocytic defense system also produce acute phase substances. Time lapse photography, using the Naessens microscope, has demonstrated the total fragmentation of certain granulocytes in AIDS patients over a twelve hour period.* This indication that the AIDS virus may affect elements of all white blood cells may explain the impossibility of restoration of the immune system by focusing primarily on the T4 lymphocyte. Anemia and diminished indices of red cell morphology may be from intracellular inclusions of organisms, but also from damaged stem cells, the progenitor of both red and white blood cells. Altered hematologic values, although non-specific, are probably the most consistent indicator of the presence of the AIDS virus.

---

*page 120

Abnormally low serum cholesterol levels are frequently noted but seldom commented on when they are found in AIDS. A relationship between low cholesterol and cancer was first noted in the Framingham study. The latter is a long term correlation of laboratory findings in a Massachussets community with the subsequent development of cardiovascular disease among the participants in the study. Below normal cholesterol levels in connection with cancer have been widely noted by the medical community, but no one seems to know just what this means.

It has been suggested that low cholesterol might be considered a marker for cancer. More likely, it indicates the presence of pleomorphic organisms, which frequently require cholesterol as an essential nutrient. Low cholesterol levels are probably a common denominator of both conditions. Another explanation for low cholesterol in the two conditions aligns with Dr. Revici's characterization of the catabolic imbalances found in AIDS and often in cancer; among their laboratory findings are acidosis, lympopenia (low white cell count) and low sterol (which includes cholesterol).

Much medical research has concentrated on the viral etiology of cancer because of virus-like particles, frequently found in cancer tissue and in the sera of leukemia patients by electron microscopy. To the frustration of those who have worked with them, these particles cannot be grown by usual virologic techniques. It appears likely that a number of these will turn out to be the viral-like spore forms of pleomorphic organisms, a classification orthodox researchers have avoided acknowledging.

In the 1960s, Dr. Firkin of the University of Sydney demonstrated that these particles were probably derived from platelets; his work was confirmed by Drs. A.M. Prince and W.R. Adams of Yale Medical School who used density gradient fractionation as their probe. The particles banded identically with platelet lysosomes (intracellular oval structures whose secretory enzymes have digestive and metabolic functions within the cell).

Under electron microscopy, these structures demonstrated an unexpected complexity, with occasional tailed forms, helical structures and nucleoid like processes, some empty and others extruding a dumbbell shaped inner particle. The longer the plasma sample stood, the more particles were found. Drs. Prince and Adams also found these particles in all plasma samples, including those from normal and healthy individuals. They concluded that the particles were virus-like but not viruses, so there has been no further interest in them in this country.

In Italy, Dr. G. Tedeschi of the University of Camerino, long an authority on cell wall deficient organisms, has repeatedly demonstrated their presence in red blood cells and also in platelets; he has grown them through their full life cycles in the proper media, and has demonstrated them by both dark field and electron microscopy.

The Naessens microscope, capable of confirming the work of Tedeschi, may put a new and solid footing under all areas of biology and also re-direct attention to the validity of Beauchamp's original microzyme work. It should recreate an interest in the mid-century research of Rife and his microscope and in the work of that also unorthodox and persecuted genius, Wilhelm Reich. The latter implicated what he called "T-bacilli" as the basis for cancer, and believed that they came from the degeneration of body protein. Anticipating the work of Wyburn-Mason, Reich also noted the presence of ameboid parasites in cancer tissue. These organisms have also been observed under the Naessens microscope.

That there can be microorganisms, originating within platelets as well as within red blod cells, is a radical departure from all standard doctrines of biology. That they can under normal circumstances be the impetus for normal cell division, suggests that their abnormal proliferation may likewise be the impetus for cancer formation. A totally new approach to the prevention and treatment of cancer may be possible. This proposition exceeds even the concepts of cell wall deficient organisms. It is not too much at variance with the wide distribution of protozoa and other parasites (including amoeba and even Pneumocystis Carinii) within almost all mammalian species; these emerge as pathogens when the defenses of the body are inadequate.

Consideration of these far out propositions evokes Hans Selye's statement that "Great progress can be made only by ideas very different from those generally accepted at the time. Unfortunately, it is literally true that the more someone sticks out his neck above the masses, the more he is likely to attract the eyes of snipers. . . . Very few fundamentally new ideas manage to by-pass the heresey stage. . . . A new concept in biology . . . is almost certain to provoke what Huxley called a 'public war dance'."

The Medical Establishment has ignored or opposed for a long time the research and the practices that are now in the wings. It will be insufficient that the urgency of the AIDS crisis may induce more researchers to be receptive to them. Possible benefits from them will continue to be unavailable to the general public unless the legal blockade of "proof of efficacy" requirements is removed from the FDA so they can be commercially developed. This is urgently needed.

25

PROFESSIONAL AND INSTITUTIONAL INTERPLAYS

More than three years of AIDS research has failed to show that anyone has ever developed AIDS-related Complex, Kaposi's sarcoma or Opportunistic Infection from the AIDS virus alone. The medical profession, placing the cart before the horse, has assumed that the AIDS virus, by attacking the T-4 lymphocytes, destroys the immune system and allows Opportunistic Infection (with which it considers Kaposi's sarcoma basically the same) and secondary viral infections, to emerge. That the AIDS virus is the precipitating co-factor (only in those whose defense systems are already inadequate, depleted or suppressed) is a concept that is slowly and reluctantly recognized or considered by researchers and clinicians.

The multi-causal etiology of AIDS has been generally ignored by the many workers and participants of the medical scene whose interests are advanced by a single agent explanation for the syndrome:

The RESEARCH TEAMS of Dr. Gallo and of Dr. Montaigner have gained renown for their brilliant work that culminated in the isolation of the AIDS virus. Their achievements will be diminished but not abolished by recognition that the AIDS virus is the frosted top of a many layered cake, but it is not the cake itself.

IMMUNOLOGISTS, astronauts of the medical space probe, have focused on depression of lymphocyte-derived cell immunity as the central derangement of AIDS. A monocausal etiology of AIDS provides a rationale for their attempts to cure AIDS by concentrating on restoration of cell mediated immunity. This is equivalent to the repair of a burned-out motor by replacing the ignition system and refilling the crank case with oil.

DERMATOLOGISTS, equally specialized as the immunologists and knowing as little general medicine and physiology, have also not perceived the broader aspects of the problem. They have failed to recognize that Kaposi's sarcoma, by itself, is not an equivalent of Opportunistic Infection, but a separate entity. Riding the immunology-cancer bandwagon, the dermatologists have been equally narrow in their treatment of Kaposi's sarcoma and their patients.

A single disease agent that just happened to have emerged within the GAY COMMUNITY, absolves its members from individual or collective responsibilities for containing or controlling the spread of AIDS, either among them or from them.

A single agent, causing disease primarily of the skin and the immune system, has enabled many of THE MEDICAL PROFESSION to avoid treating its victims. An acceptance of its multi-faceted microbial cause and wide systems involvement will imply a broader basis of therapy than is currently practiced; modifying many previously unquestioned aspects of scientific medicine, it will open avenues of therapy which have so far been confined to Health Oriented Medicine.

GOVERNMENTAL HEALTH AGENCIES, coordinating, directing and funding the majority of AIDS projects, have been able to point with pride to their success in solving the major problem of AIDS—its cause. Previous dissatisfactions and criticism of these agencies (especially the National Institutes of Health) have been muted but they will flare anew with public recognition that spotlighting the AIDS virus as the cause of AIDS is an incomplete and misleading solution of a complicated issue. The Centers for Disease Control (CDC) will, understandably, not be happy to add further complexities and complications to their already wide activities and responsibilities. The FDA will be unhappy as multi-causal aspects of AIDS imply possible benefits or relevance of biologic and other therapies of alternative and Health Oriented Medicine which the FDA has long opposed or removed from the market. Attention directed to them will lead to a renewed public interest in FDA function and policy.

Although Scientific Medicine is the accepted standard of all Western nations, political and sociologic factors largely determine the type of medicine available for the general population in each country. Ironically, it is within the United States, where the AIDS problem is the most urgent, that many of the approaches and therapies that appear of benefit in the treatment of AIDS, are legally unavailable. In short, the AIDS problem and its resolutions are intimately tied to the political and institutional framework of the Medical Establishment, with which all Scientific Medicine is interwoven.

26

SCIENTISM—A DISTORTION OF SCIENCE

Authority is the underpinning of civilization and man's inborn deference to authority the basis by which rulers maintain power and prestige. The explosion of knowledge and the intellectual ferment of the Renaissance loosened Western man's unquestioned deference and faith in ecclesiastical and feudal authority but transferred it relatively unchanged to science and reason.

With few exceptions, major advances in traditional medicine have come from basic observation of the patient and his disease and from the reasoning of individual physicians, not from the direction and consensus of committees or authority. Within the laboratory, the objectivity of scientific methodology is generally maintained, but within the institutions that comprise the Medical Establishment, there has evolved a motivating philosophy, inherently bureaucratic, which is mislabeled "science" but is better termed "scientism".

Scientism is the faith that all phenomena can be reduced to physical and measurable terms and that all problems of human health and medical care can be solved by scientific method, laboratory investigation and legislative control. Medical scientism blots all that cannot be explained in terms of existing knowledge. It refuses to accept the principles and practices of any therapy

133

not sanctioned by custom or academic approval. Scientism, poorly recognizing that what is perceived as truth changes with time and increasing knowledge, considers scientific truth to be absolute, to be preserved by authority and protected from those who would question or modify it. The great Osler (Sir William) is reported to have once startled his medical students by stating "Gentlemen, half of all that I have taught you is wrong; unfortunately, I don't know which half it is."

Scientism accumulates data and maintains establishment amenities; its reverential attitude toward medical authority permeates and influences our legislative bodies and courts of law.

The rigidity and narrowness of the scientific ego has been outlined by Kubie and other psychologic investigators. The strong identification of the individual scientist with the scientific establishment leads him to construe a challenge to the institution as an attack upon his personal faith, and thus he vehemently and emotionally resists that challenge by every available means.

Medical scientism ignores the empiric approaches of traditional medicine. It discounts clinical observation as being "anecdotal" and enshrines as the sole basis for valid medicial judgement, statistical analysis, double blind studies and the prevailing consensus of opinion. It relies on the use of animals for drug efficacy and seldom accepts that animals (especially the mouse) are not identical to humans. Had the guinea pig instead of the mouse been used in early Penicillin experiments, the specific convulsive reaction of guinea pigs to Penicillin would have canceled any further research on it. Were penicillin recently discovered, it would not easily or quickly pass current FDA regulations for effectiveness and safety. The majority of our important drugs have been empirically developed and the major advances of traditional medicine have been generally ignored or opposed by the Medical Establishment of the time.

Scientism uses knowledge only within a programmed

framework, opposes innovation, conforms to the past and combines with the bureaucratic propensities of our major medical institutions.

Scientism is probably best illustrated by Chlorozone, patented in the 1960s as an effective method of water purification, derived from a special electrolytic processing of salt water. The active ingredients of Chlorozone are presumably ozone, chloride ions and other oxydizing products of the saline solution. Chlorozone has been used successfullly as a disinfectant for swimming pools (it is non irritating to the eyes and mucous membranes, and does not bleach materials); it is a highly effective germicide against both viruses and bacteria.

In the early 1970s, Chlorozone, used in the water supply of Zakynthos (a Greek village), dramatically reduced an epidemic of infectious hepatitis.

More importantly, Chlorozone was extensively investigated there for its medical applications. It was administered to over 200 volunteers in areas of degenerative disease otherwise poorly treated; its topical, oral, and intravenously administered effects were impressive, well documented and published by Ross Gwynn in "Bioelectrolysis in Man". Beneficial effects were noted in almost all areas, particularly in the relief of pain (outstanding in burns and in cancer); there was prolongation of life and comfort in terminal cancer patients and restoration of function in many chronically ill individuals. These included patients with vascular disease, arthritis and neurologic conditions (it appeared especially beneficial in multiple sclerosis and parkinsonism). Full records were kept and these were attested by reputable physicians (including an associate professor of Orthopedics at the University of Athens Medical School). These reports were consistant with Chlorozone's beneficial effects previously in Viet Nam where it had been used by a medical unit in the treatment of civilian war casualties For over a decade, on the basis of the Greek study, and despite affidavits of MDs and patients, the inventor has vainly attempted to obtain a patent for the possible medical values of chlorozone. Without a patent, there can be no adequate medical investigation or commercial development of any product. The Patent Office has repeatedly turned down patent applications for Chlorozone by the rationale that the inventor's explanation for its medical effects are not sufficiently scientific and do not align to prevailing medical opinions. This bureaucratic scientism would be unfortunate at any time, but especially now when Chlorozone might be of value in treating patients with AIDS. In a limited study, it has relieved pain from edematous Kaposi lesions of the feet, increased white blood cell counts, and appeared to contribute to the well being of patients. Its beneficial general effects appear to follow other modalities (Ozone, Hydrochloric Acid therapy, and ultraviolet irradiation of blood) that increase the delivery of oxygen (and probably its utilization) to the tissues.

Huntington Beach, Ca. 92646

Dear Dr. Brown:

As per our telephone conversation, I am pleased to advise you of my personal investigation of the Chlorozone medical studies run in Greece during the period I was there (1968-70), and apparently after I left.

I was first aware of Chlorozone's medical effects when an electronic team from Italy arrived at my office with three of the five men continuously vomiting and diarrheal from bad fish they had eaten on the ferry boat from Italy to Greece. When each of the men affected had drunk a glass of Chlorozone solution, their discomfort and symptoms subsided totally within minutes. They had subsequently refused to go into the field to do their work unless each had a bottle of Chlorozone "just in case."

My interest was aroused by this incident, and more so when I heard of some of the remarkable results of Chlorozone therapy in a variety of medical conditions. Among the cases I investigated was a woman with multiple sclerosis, approximately 35 years old, who for several months had been totally confined to bed in the fetal position. After several weeks of chlorozone therapy, she could straighten up, speak almost coherently, and ultimately was able to sit at table with her family for dinner.

Another instance I recall, although I did not witness, was an outbreak of hepatitis on the island of Zakynthos, which subsided after a chlorozone generator was installed there in the water supply.

On a personal basis, my lifelong suseptibility to colds, sore throats and chronic coughs subsided when I began gargling with Chlorozone and expectorating it through my mouth from sniffing it through my nose. My sore throats would disappear within the hour.

Needless to say, I was most impressed by the results of Chlorozone and the various Greek doctors that I met who were using it for various maladies. There was one doctor, whose name I can not recall, who was using it at the Athens burn center to treat third degree burns. His patients immediately seemed to be out of pain after chlorozone was topically applied.

I hope the above sketchy information is of value. I will be happy to provide more details, should you wish.

sincerely yours,

Edgar Benditzky

Edgar Benditzky

25 Nov. 1985

27

THE MEDICAL ESTABLISHMENT

The Medical Establishment is a loose web of Academia (schools, hospitals and research institutes), professional associations, governmental health and regulatory agencies, health foundations and the pharmaceutical industry. Allied with Scientific Medicine, the Medical Establishment has achieved prominence, prestige and power from the medical advances of this century, but it is increasingly bureaucratic, conservative and intolerant of approaches and practices outside its boundaries. Members of the medical profession, by their possession of medical degrees, are considered uniquely qualified for positions of authority and counsel; they staff Academia, serve in the government, disburse funds, control professional publications, instruct the news media, and advise legislatures and industry. They are the thread that unites all factions of the Establishment and like adversary lawyers in court, they move easily and interchangeably through competing, and at times opposing, areas of activity; their homogeneity of outlook and training provides liaison and leadership in maintaining institutional and establishment control against outside assaults. Rules of the game over-ride personal involvement, and the passage of time sees roles reversed or interchanged. A familiar scenario is the musical chairs interchange of personnel among Academia, government, industry and foundations.

Oriental and primitive cultures absorb and bond the individual to the fabric of family, with allegiances extending outwards to tribe, government and cosmos; social stability and order stem from the individual's identity with his niche in the Cosmic-All. Although stretched, the fabric of the old order is still relatively intact in the Orient, but in the West, man has set himself adrift from the demands and protection of family or religion and from faith in government. In his search for identity and meaning, he fills the void by identification with the institutions which he creates. His belief that their activities have purpose extends beyond rationalization or intellect, rendering him immune to self-criticism and blind to personal accountability; bureaucratic qualifications and expediency too often take precedence over morality or ethics.

Within the Medical Establishment, orthodoxy is maintained by control of medical education, research funding and professional publications. What is not popular is seldom funded or published. The Medical Establishment credo "Don't rock the boat" attempts to preserve the mutually rewarding and protective system of balances created among its individual institutions over the years.

Like Toynbee's civilizations, institutions arise from a specific need, thrive on challenge and decrease in flexibility and vision as they enter middle age. This applies to the majority of medical institutions, which, like individuals, do not self-destruct with age but expend their energies to maintain their accumulated power and resources. Churchill's remark that he did not become prime minister to preside over the liquidation of the British Empire applies equally to the determination of the Medical Establishment to preserve its carefully built institutions.

Changes, however, are occuring as previously comfortable

alliances among the institutions are loosening. There is a growing unease that the old approaches and rules may not apply and that previous guideposts and maps may not be pertinent to the altered landscape of today. It is likely that the stresses and strains imposed by AIDS across all medical institutions will profoundly affect the structure of the Medical Establishment. As medical institutions, respectively controlling major aspects of medical research and of medical practice, the National Institutes of Health and the Food and Drug Administration are the most likely to be affected.

28

THE NATIONAL INSTITUTES
OF HEALTH (NIH)

The National Institutes of Health (NIH), the government medical research center and the major funding agency for medical research throughout the country, is a bastion of conservatism that has poured billions of dollars down the avenues of orthodoxy and scientific fashion. Its guidelines, like military rules and regulations, protect the conventional while discouraging originality or independence. By its control of funding (the life blood of research), it has disseminated and perpetuated the conservatism of its advisors and consultants, who are drawn almost exclusively from teaching and research centers.

The NIH embodies the strengths and weaknesses of our major research institutions. It has the prestige and superb physical facilities of a top governmental organization, but also the burden of proximity to Congress. Responsive to the temper of the general public, our legislators are increasingly critical of the poor performance of the NIH and of government funded institutions in solvng our major medical and health problems.

Some of the problem is semantics. It is poorly understood that basic science, which is fundamental to medical research, is the pursuit of knowledge only for its own sake. Like Mount

Everest, it is there, but its challenges and satisfactions, although they may be rationalized, cannot be justified in terms of any immediate benefit to mankind. Medical research belongs not to medicine, which is concerned with the treatment of the sick individual, but to science which is concerned with the increase and systemization of knowledge. The attempt to solve health and medical problems belongs to the realm of applied science; this depends not only on knowledge from basic research but also on the wisdom and intuition of its clinicians. Physicians who posssess these qualities are increasingly rare in Academia, so research institutions are usually dominated by committeee approval, academic conformity, targeted programs and bureaucratic regulations.

Concepts of the biologic unity which underlies and maintains our health are seldom noted. Medical researchers use the patient primarily to demonstrate findings derived from the laboratory, although historically the major advances of medicine have been initiated by clinical observation with verification by clinical trials and laboratory studies. Academia's orientation to research and specialization has produced few researchers capable of innovative thought or independent action outside their specialized areas.

The inadequacies of the NIH have been most evident in cancer research. A major interest when the NIH was founded in the 1940s was the role of nutrition in cancer, but this was totally discarded as chemotherapy and virology permeated and dominated research thinking. Money, talent and time were expended over three decades in a search for cancer's viral cause and chemical cure. Although scientific knowledge increased astronomically, the major advancements in cancer therapy came as refinements of diagnosis, surgery, radiation and chemotherapy. The viral etiology of cancer, first suggested by Rous's work at Rockefeller Institute in the 1920s, culminated in the 1980s work of Gallo at NIH with the Human T-Cell Leukemia Virus (HTLV), whose strain III is currently implicated in AIDS.

Pertinent to the current stalemate in AIDS research are some past comments by prominent medical researchers. One of Dr. Hans Selye's deep concerns was the danger to medical science of superspecialization. IN VIVO, a 1967 collection of his lectures, addresses the issue by pleading for a return to "old fashioned supra-nuclear biology of simple observation at the biologic level, rather than high technology and planned research . . . which limits breadth by zeroing in too sharply on individual targets. . . . Few scientists maintain a working familiarity with many fields. . . . We shall always need at least a few general practitioners of medical research, men whose minds are open to the many things that come their way. We shall depend upon them in research just as we shall always require general practitioners of clinical medicine who can look at the patient as a whole."

Nobel prize winner, Dr. Albert Szent Gyorgi, in the foreword to IN VIVO affirms Dr. Selye's convictions: "The molecular level is but one of the many levels of organization, and what we call life is an integral of all functions and reactions. The integrated level of the whole is the most complex and also the most difficult field of research. It is this level which also has all the charm and whimsicalness of life. To approach it we must be in direct personal contact with it and not only observe it by watching pointers of involved hardware. We must use all our senses, including two outdated instruments: eyes and brains."

The late Dr. Colin Macleod of Rockefeller Institute commented that "We are all aware of fads and fashions in research, which constitute one of the banes of the scientific life. An investigator announces a significant discovery, whereupon squads of research workers abandon what they were doing and move in to mop up. This common tactic stems from psychological insecurity, the fear of being alone in the ocean of scientific ignorance, with all the self-doubts this engenders. Much better to be hunting with the pack, or, as it is put 'to be in the forefront of scientific advances'."

Sir F. MacFarlane Burnet, the great Australian immunologist has commented: "The intellectual attraction of microbiology and immunology today is at the level of molecular biology and biochemical genetics. . . . It is a magnificant continuing achievement and it has no bearing whatever on human needs. . . . Human biology in the broadest sense is the science of the future. . . . It is urgent that an increasing proportion of men with first rate capacity move away from the laboratories to the direct and practical, but still scholarly application of biological science to men and their problems".

29

THE FOOD AND DRUG ADMINISTRATION (FDA)

The FDA, probably the most powerful and essential institution of the Medical Establishment, has probably been the most demoralized, inept and excoriated of any regulatory agency within the government. Under the jurisdiction of eight separate congressional subcommittees, it had in a three year period the unenviable record of one hundred unfavorable investigations by Congress.

Founded for the purpose of achieving purity and safety in our food and medicines, the FDA has never achieved its goals. By its control over the manufacture and availability of all drugs and medical equipment, it controls medical practice and medical research to a degree unequaled by any other institution. Functioning virtually as a National Department of Medicine, its current role far exceeds the original intent of Congress.

In 1906, in an attempt to curb the rampant evils of the food industry, a Food and Drug Act was passed 63-4 by the Senate and 241-7 by the House of Representatives. Backed by the AMA, the Federated Women's Clubs of America, the Consumer's League, the American Public Health Association, the Patrons of Husbandry, the Federated Labor Organizations, state health agencies and a majority of the concerned public, the Act appeared to assure the safety of the Nation's food and drugs.

145

The Bureau of Chemistry, established as an outgrowth of the Agriculture Department in the 1860s and long active in advocating food and drug legislation, was designed to collect and submit evidence of violations to the Department of Justice for prosecution. Harvey W. Wiley, MD, its director, was a man of more integrity than political sophistication or tact. His frontal assaults on the windmills of the liquor, Coca Cola, milling and food industries unhorsed him in six years. Opposed to saccharine as a sugar substitute, he reportedly lost the support of President Theodore Roosevelt who used it for weight control. Industry, which had failed to prevent the passage of the Food and Drug Act, effectively worked through the political bureaucracy of Washington to subvert it. Wiley resigned when an emasculated Bureau of Chemistry was transferred to its arch-rival, the Department of Agriculture; thereafter and therein, it languished in the role of an advisory group only.

Widely publicized was Wiley's use of "The Poison Squad", a group of young volunteers who took part in a long-range evaluation of a diet containing whatever food additives were being studied. The tests, conducted over a period of ten years, demonstrated the toxicity of chemicals previously considered safe (including boric acid, the salicylates, benzoic acid and the benzoites, sulfur dioxide, the sulfites, formaldehyde, copper sulfate and saltpeter). Meticulously conducted and monitored, the reports were widely featured in the press, but so strong was the pressure brought against them by the chemical industry that many of the reports were suppressed even from governmental printing. The validity of these experiments was subsequently confirmed so that all the foregoing chemicals are banned from food except for sulfur dioxide, and that is currently the focus of much documented criticism.

The issues in which Wiley was involved are again matters of public concern and his warnings of the dangers from adulterated food and chemicals is as pertinent today as in his time.

The FDA emerged from obscurity within the Agriculture Department in 1938 when Congress passed the Food, Drug and Cosmetics Act in response to more than one hundred deaths which resulted from faultily manufactured Sulfanilamide. This legislation required that new drugs pass safety tests and that the relevant data be submitted to the government for clearance prior to licensing.

In 1962, Thalidomide, a sedative for expectant mothers, caused congenital deformities in several thousand British and German infants. The tragedy was averted in the United States because the drug had not been administratively cleared through the FDA. This narrow escape indelibly changed the course of the FDA and of American medicine.

In a burst of good intentions, politics, and misguided scientism, the Kefauver-Harris Amendment to the 1938 Act was pushed through Congress. This gave police powers to the FDA to make and enforce decisions on drug safety autonomously; more crucially, proof of efficacy, in addition to that of safety, was mandated for drug licensing. This measure introduced chaos into an already confused agency. Proof of efficacy, like proof of virtue, is difficult at best to obtain, dependent largely on the eye (and the emotional and mental biases) of the beholder. It is the means by which the FDA influences the entire medical field with iron control and final decision-making over the manufacturing, testing, and distribution of drugs. The FDA acquired power across the field of medicine that even the American Medical Association does not possess. This was further augmented in 1975 when the FDA acquired the further power to control all aspects of medical devices and equipment on the basis of effectiveness as well as safety.

American medicine lacks many good products and therapies available in other countries, as the majority of FDA decisions concerning drugs are made by bureaucrats who have never practiced medicine. By generally refusing to acknowledge or accept foreign research, to allow drug combinations, or many biologic products, the FDA protects itself from the intrusion of ideas and products it cannot understand or control. Oriented to large industry, the FDA has totally eliminated small innovative pharmaceutical houses by imposing impossible financial and testing demands on them. The minimum expenditure of twenty million dollars and ten years for any new product ensures that only the large drug companies, which produce almost exclusively highly profitable and generally expensive products, can compete. Only one in two hundred drugs that are submitted to the FDA for licensing are approved. By present day FDA standards, it would be difficult and probably impossible to introduce Aspirin, Penicillin, Insulin, or electrocardiographic equipment into production.

The agency's close ties to industry, from which FDA officials are frequently drawn, and to which they return following government service, have produced FDA leniency toward safety standards for many industry products. This conflict between public safety and industrial profits has been most evident within the food industry. While the FDA has rigidly applied its "presumption of guilt until proven innocent" formula to judging the effectiveness of medical materials, it has usually assumed that all chemical additves to food are harmless until their health dangers are conclusively proved, usually by the companies which produce them.

The mandates given by Congress to the FDA have been so broad and the potential for power so tempting that the bureaucratic monster thus created has almost foundered in trying to carry out the impossible duties it has been given. Overseeing a budget which rose from $5 million in 1955 to $279 million in 1977, it has the responsibility for passing on the merits of over $200 billion worth of products each year. The FDA sprawls across the center of government, and by its Byzantine internal politics, has threatened and harassed employees who have directed attention to its inadequacies. It has worn out those within and from outside who have attempted to reform it, and has expended its energies in scientism and a bureaucratic expansion of power at the expense of common sense and service.

The closet skeletons, peccadillos, and derelictions of the FDA surface to public attention with each investigation or report. Among the many books published concerning the FDA, the most authoritative and explicit have been "DMSO, the Persecuted Drug" by the late Pat McGrady, "Eating may be Dangerous to your Health" by FDA scientist Jacqueline Verrett, "Power Inc." by Mintz and Cohen, and "The Chemical Feast" by James Turner. When the latter was published, Time Magazine said "It may well be the most devastating critique of a United States Government agency ever issued".

Traditionally, the art of medicine has been advanced by the observations and practical clinical experience of patient-oriented physicians. Today, the increasing regimentation and conformity imposed on physicians by the Medical Establishment, and especially the FDA, discourage innovation. The spector of malpractice suits and of persecution hangs over any physician who is brave enough to try publicly old drugs for new uses or to administer therapies not sanctioned by the consensus of practicing physicians. For almost all chronic and degenerative diseases, and especially AIDS and cancer, the adjunctive therapies that are of potential benefit are almost all resolutely opposed by the FDA.

The only hope for achieving a more effective FDA is to reestablish its original purpose of testing and maintaining the safety and purity of our food and drugs. It must be relieved of its unmanageable and impossible burden of determining and assuring effectiveness of drugs and devices.

The FDA should follow a simple rating system for effectiveness and safety. Effectiveness would fall into one of three categoriess "Effectiveness Unconditionally Proved", "Effectiveness conditionally demonstrated", and "Effectiveness undetermined". Safety could also be categorized in the same manner and the appropriate designation then affixed to all products or containers. Judgement of the effectiveness of any medical product or device should not be vested in any governmental agency or institutions but should be returned to the province of the individual physician. Freedom of choice for medical materials, therapy and methods must be put on the same footing as civil liberties and as vigorously protected. The processes and powers by which the FDA has functioned as policeman, prosecuting attorney and judge of medical practice must be amended, and only legislative action can accomplish this.

In the final analysis, only a concerned citizenry, exerting power through their elected representatives in Congress, can achieve the needed reform of the FDA. Only then can American medicine achieve its full potential.

30

CONFLICTS AND POWER PLAYS (THERE SHOULD BE A LAW?)

Health and medical conflicts, widely reported in the media, smoulder and periodically erupt across the American landscape. They usually involve large industry versus the environment, the food and drug industries versus the consumer, the Medical Establishment versus change and the medical profession versus competition.

The public increasingly questions the credibility and authority of previously unquestioned institutions, including government, industry and science; the motivations, philosophy and ethics of medical practice are now considered reasonable subjects for public discussion and review.

Environmental catastrophies and health disasters from chemicals released into the air, ground and our water supplies have vindicated the early and unheeded warnings of environmentalists and ecologists, beginning with Rachael Carson. Many of the health issues today can be seen as large industry versus the environment with government as intermediary, attempting to control dangerous industrial practices without throttling productivity and economic growth.

Loosely controlled agricultural and food processing practices and the manipulations of our dietary and pharmaceutical habits by the advertising media, have been generally for the welfare of the pharmaceutical and food industries and not the consumer.

In the absence of a governmental consumer agency, concern for our nutritional safety and health has stemmed primarily from the health movement and from Congress, on whom the ultimate responsibility for public health policy depends. The landmark recommendations of the 1975 Senate Select Committee on Nutrition and Human Needs were more influenced by the health movement and by individuals than by the Medical Establishment. Dependency on foundation, government and industry grants has compromised the intellectual objectivity of medical researchers who shrink from controversy and are often reluctant to acknowledge industrial responsibility toward population health.

In Congress, the obvious medical concerns are cost and availability of medical care; the latter has been generally viewed as a commodity service like the railroads—to be regulated, and if necessary, subsidized. Financial and administrative problems of health and medical care are based on the premise that adequate care can only be provided by the Medical Establishment and should be delivered only by the the medical profession. Congress has had neither the time nor the incentive to investigate the substance of medicine or the performance of the medical profession. In the field of unorthodox medical therapy (and especially in the areas of cancer), successive Congressional investigations have accomplished little but to waste the taxpayer's money and the legislator's time. They have primarily demonstrated that the central issue is the failure of the individuals and the therapies investigated to conform to authority and current medical practices. From the presumption that all reports by individual physicians are suspect and that neither the patient nor the individual doctor can judge effectiveness of therapy, hundreds of cases of successfully treated patients have been dismissed as "anecdotal" and thereby eliminated from medical consideration;

positive results which cannot be ignored, are dismissed under the label "spontaneous remission".

The Medical Establishment and the health industry (hospitals, nursing homes, clinics, health care personnel and the providers of health and medical products) are coalitions of interest whose individual and continued welfare depends on a strong medical profession. They are united in their concern against external infringement and internal irregularities of medical practice that compete with or lessen their share of money available for health and medical care.

Much of today's medical turmoil results from the Medical Establishment's resistance to change. Older concepts of Health Oriented Medicine have been generally submerged by technology and chemical pharmacology (based on medical research) even as these have exceeded the ability of the individual, or even the government, to afford them. The Health Movement, supporting alternative systems of health and medical care and advocating freedom of choice for the patient, has followed the precepts of Dr. Benjamin Rush. That well known physician of the Colonial era, and signer of the Declaration of Independence, opposed official recognition of any one system of medicine, much as the Constitution forbade the establishment of a state religion.

Non-conforming physicians are at frequent odds with the Medical Establishment. They threaten the membership and strength of the AMA and its associated organizations; their usually health-oriented practices decrease the elitism and monopolies of specialties; their lessened emphasis on chemical pharmaceuticals compete with the drug industry. Their preventive medical approaches, closely linked to the naturopathic tendencies of extra-medical health disciplines, are noticeably less dependant upon hospital based technology. This secularization of medicine threatens all segments of the Medical Establishment; the FDA, protected by its governmental status, has always been vigilant in prosecuting non-conformist practitioners.

In the 1960's the FDA (aided by the American Medical Association) successfully eliminated a growing professional interest in the nutritionally based Turkel therapy for Down's Syndrome. Its unsuccessful drive in 1975 to limit the availability of vitamins, minerals and other nutritional supplements to the general public was part of a larger Establishment drive against nutritional and naturopathic therapies. In the cancer field the FDA has been more effective than the AMA or the American Cancer Society in curtailing the use of alternative cancer therapies.

The use of chelation therapy, by threatening conventional concepts of vascular disease and affecting the practice of cardiology and vascular surgery, inevitably produced the revocation of Dr. Ray Ever's license to practice medicine in Louisiana. It also led to two attempts to prosecute him in Alabama. These attacks on the foremost practitioner and advocate of chelation therapy thereby served as warning to physicians of the difficulties in using and advocating unsanctioned medical therapies. Dr. Robert Harris of Connecticut was placed on 5 years probation and fined $5,000 for using chelation therapy in his practice. In New Jersey and Pennyslvania, Dr. Peter Marco lost his license for successfully treating vascular disease with a substance closely related to Gerovital (the controversial Roumanian anti-aging therapy). In Virginia, the medical license of Dr. Thomas Roberts was revoked by the state medical board for including nutritional regimes in far advanced cancer patients. The story has been repeated across the country with dismaying frequency; physicians have lost their licenses, not because of malpractice but because their philosophy and approaches have not conformd to authority and the practices of a majority of physicians.

When innovations within medical practice cannot be contained by restricting the availability of materials, the crushing financial burden of legal defense against unlimited and repeated governmental prosecution has been usually successful. The FDA eliminated Glyoxalide, a homeopathic material which was effective in viral infections and cancer, only after Dr. William Koch, its originator, had been jailed and had spent nearly a million dollars in four court cases against charges of mislabeling his product.

Almost all legal cases involving health or medical issues today are variations of Establishment manipulations to restrict the fields of health and medicine. The mid-century success of wonder drugs and hospital based technology appeared to confirm the assumption that only the medical profession is competent to provide health care, and to justify the long history of Establishment prosecution against herbalists, native Indian practitioners, nutritionists, naturopaths, homeopaths, chiropractors and other lesser breeds.

Treatment of specific disease does not guarantee health, which is the proper functioning of all aspects of an individual. Health oriented practices, primarily directed at improving all functions of the body (and secondarily the treatment of specific disease) encourage patients to share responsibility and take an active role in their own treatment. This has made the legal distinction between health care and medical care increasingly difficult to define legally.

The treatment of AIDS focuses many of the public's dissatisfactions with the services provided by the Medical Establishment. As in cancer, the exorbitant cost of major medical care excludes many who most need it; the rapidly increasing number of AIDS cases is straining medical facilities in the locations hardest hit by the epidemic.

The 1970s attempt by the Medical Establishment, primarily represented by the FDA, to classify all nutritional products as drugs and thus available only by prescription, was defeated by a grass roots response from the population to Congress. The coalition of major health movement organizations, health oriented physicians and concerned individuals demonstrated to

Congress their increasing strength as a political counterpoise to the Medical Establishment.

Although this attempt failed, the Medical Establishment (primarily the AMA and the FDA) succeeded in another power struggle whose unfortunate results affect the clinical practices of many health oriented physicians and by extension, their patients.

Adrenal cortex extract (ACE), widely used as replacement therapy in Addison's Disease (adrenal insufficiency), comparable to the use of insulin in diabetes, was notable for few side effects or toxicity. In 1964, the AMA'S council on Drug Evaluation had declared: "No synthetic substance posseses all the effects of a potent cortical extract". The increasing use of adrenal cortical extract (ACE) by health oriented physicians for the treatment of hypoglycemia (low blood sugar), and in severe allergies (also poorly treated conventionally) became an issue comparable to chelation therapy today. That the use of ACE was widely promoted by the health movement and used by health oriented physicians was apparently sufficient reason for eliminating it from medical availability. The AMA ignored its previous Council findings and by its opposition (comparable to its current opposition to chelation therapy) backed the FDA's removal of ACE from the market.

Today, the adrenal insufficiency of AIDS patients, characterized by hypoglycemia, hypotension (low blood pressure) and other clinical indications of adrenal depletion is seldom noted and poorly treated by the synthetic steroids that are available. Their imbalanced and eventually deleterious effects, either pro-inflammatory or anti-inflammatory, when used alone are increasingly evident. It is rather certain that the FDA and the AMA blotted out an extremely good product that is now urgently needed.

That AIDS is even partially amenable to health oriented approaches provides a push to the medical treatment pendulum.

The far limit of technology and chemical pharmaceuticals has possibly been reached and there may now be a beginning return to more biologic and affordable health-oriented medical care. If so, it may emphasize that strong defenses of health are the responsibility of the individual and not of medical science; drugs and technology may more widely be viewed as augmenting, but not replacing, proper nutrition, mental attitudes, life styles and balanced ecology within our bodies and our environment.

As pertinent to AIDS as to cancer is a landmark article published in the July 1984 issue of the prestigious Annals of Internal Medicine, by Dr. Barrie Cassileth and her group at the University of Pennyslvania. Entitled "Contemporary Unorthodox Treatments in Cancer Medicine, A Study of Patients, Treatments, and Practitioners", it addresses the question of why, in a period of advanced technology are patients, attracted to therapeutic alternatives outside the Medical Establishment. It documents extensive interviews with 356 cancer patients on unconventional regimes and with a similar group on orthodox therapy. It notes that statistically the unorthodox group was better educated, 40% of them had abandoned conventional therapy entirely after adopting alternative regimes, and that the costs of most unconventional therapies are modest in comparison to orthodox therapy. It states that patients are attracted to therapeutic alternatives that reflect social emphasis on personal responsibility, nutrition and environmental ecology and that move away from what they view as deficiencies of conventional medical care.

The article notes that although few alternative regimes are identical, most of them include therapeutic combinations derived from special diets and nutrients, vitamins, minerals, enzymes, detoxification procedures, oxidative measures, exercise, immunostimulatory regimes, homeopathy, herbals and other botanical products, cell therapy, and psychologic and spiritual regimens. The authors comment on the many patients with a wide range of chronic illnesses, as well as healthy persons who use these alternative programs in the hope of preventing disease. The study reports that patients receiving alternative care do not generally conform to the stereotype of uneducated terminally ill patients who have exhausted conventional treatment. It notes that although some unorthodox practitioners might qualify as quacks and charlatans, many are well trained, few charge high fees and most appear to believe in the validity of their work. The authors comment that contemporary alternatives are long term, lifestyle-oriented options that exist within a broad view of health and personal responsibility. They feel that as the health care and economic implications of unorthodox therapies are vast, they are unlikely to be readily discarded.

The recurrent attempts to provide legislation to protect our aging population from wasting money on "unproven" health and medical therapies are laudable in intent and deplorable in their implications. They compare to the well-intentioned 18th Amendment to the Constitution that in the 1920s attempted to protect the public from the ills of alcohol by prohibiting its possession or use for any purpose other than medical. Despite its admirable aim, prohibition was a resoundng and expensive failure in all areas of enactment.

Trying to protect our older citizens from mistakes of judgement by requiring proof of efficacy for all health and medical products and practices is dangerous. It would deliver to the Medical Establishment a weapon against all health-oriented therapies, both within medicine and in the health fields. Attempts to enforce total conformity in these areas could be disastrous for the individual and for society.

31

APPENDICEAL INCLUSIONS

Although the supplementary chapters presented here may appear to be left overs, their relationships to the preceding chapters are too pertinent to exclude them.

The acupuncture address by Dr. Smith should probably have been included in my chapter "Dimensions of Energy" but its factual material as well as its broad insights on AIDS justifies its presentation as a separate chapter.

The chapters on Vitamin D and on Dr. de Sousa (iron metabolism) may appear extraneous but illustrate the dispersal of the FDA'S energy and manpower in focusing on the elusive proof of efficacy when it should be focused on safety. The forced medication of our food, specifically our milk and our bread by ergasterol and iron respectively, is long overdue for evaluation. It is urgent that the relationships of these substances to all degenerative disease, and especially the therapeutic use of iron in AIDS and cancer, be reviewed.

I have included Max Gerson, the neglected but foremost nutritional resaarcher-clinician of the recent past to emphasize the common nutritional basis of Scientific and Health Oriented Medicine. Interest within the health field and among AIDS patients justifies the chapter on Macrobiotics.

I have expanded the references to Staphage Lysate and ul-traviolet irradiation of blood as therapeutic adjuncts in cancer and AIDS. This is directly due to my long personal and clinical interest in the former, and recent clinical experience (limited but sometimes gratifying) with the latter.

32

ACUPUNCTURE AND AIDS

(Excerpts from a 1984 speech by Michael Smith, MD., Director of the Acupuncture Clinic, Lincoln Hospital, NYC.)

We are primarily a city-supported drug abuse clinic, seeing approximately 300 patients daily, mostly with drug or alcohol related problems. Most of our sixty some AIDS cases are not drug related but are young men from lower Manhattan who come up here on their own.

There are several paradigms for how acupuncture works: one is that it improves the balances of body functions. We often use the same acupuncture point for treating low blood pressure as we do for high blood pressure and the same point for low as for high thyroid. Another way is to say that acupuncture improves body vitality.

Improving the immune system relates primarily to the respiratory and digestive systems, so many of the problems encountered in Chinese medicine refer to the lung and also the skin and to what we call "upper respiratory function". They look at this lung function and ask what type of imbalance is present. Is it from too little Yang (protective fire) or of defective Yin? One way of describing AIDS is to say that these patients do not have enough lung tone in the body and skin; when there is no tone, they lose body secretions, primarily through sweat (both daytime and at night) and they are vulnerable to outside problems which manifest in what we call "empty lung infections".

It is easy to show which persons have a vulnerability to AIDS by looking at the muscle tone of their paraspinous muscles from C-7 to T-5 and at the actual curvature of the back where the bones are tighter and more protective (possessing more Yang). This is not only diagnostic but directs us to treatment points which are in the upper back. (when it is chilly, we cover the upper back as we need to cover where this protective capacity works. This is basic to our understanding of acupuncture points; we use all posterior points; some are over the trapezius but most are related to the spinal column and smaller muscles.

Our first patient had definitely borderline psychotic aspects to his illness (which I was familiar with as psychiatry was my original field) with no ego defense . . . all these are lousy words but do describe a certain pattern of behavior . . . as the usual psychiatric patients improve, they have what we call psychiatric or personality scarring, but AIDS patients do not have this . . . it is as though it is a part of the total body phenomena.

AIDS patients are vulnerable and suggestible to a tremendous degree and this makes them easy to work with as they are congenial and interested in working to help themselves . . . but they are equally congenial to twenty five other situations and will want to try them all. These patients are not unlike cancer patients. AIDS patients should get mad more often and should not be dependant on the groups that emphasize dying but should be more active in their own behalf. A psychotherapist friend of mine who has interviewed several hundred AIDS patients reports that they just cannot get mad or react or reject their own negativity; these people are just vulnerable to all problems. You have to admit that AIDS comes from out of our society so you also have to treat the society itself. This might not be fair but illnesses are part of our social complexes.

Our clinic makes no effort to be a diagnostic center for AIDS and we have no interest in trying to be the sole treatment for these patients. Some of them have rejected all other treatments but that is their privilege. We might disagree with some of the treatments they are on but we do not use these patients as ping pong balls. If you have a strong person here and a strong person there with a suggestive patient in the middle, you can go on forever with each of you pulling on the patient and this just makes the patient worse. So many people want to give them advice and as they are very suggestible, this can be both good or bad. Even if they do well, many of them just drift off to something else and you don't see them until they have gotten into trouble again.

The other points we use for AIDS are those that improve digestive function. You want to have food that is easy on the digestive system; food that is already broken down. Other conditions relate to this. Politicians running around a lot have what is called "empty fire" and they need a lot of raw foods and juices to balance this out.

We began treating AIDS almost by accident. In December '82 we saw a man who had generalized pains and aches over his body, nightsweats and temperature; he was sort of confused and his T-cell ratio was 0.3. He told me he had AIDS and we didn't even know what that was supposed to be. This was to our advantage as we had to apply Chinese medicine and were free from the headaches of conventional thinking had we known what AIDS was supposed to be.

Acupuncture definitely improves T-cell ratios. Our first patient went from 0.3 to 2.3 in three months and he has done well, functions professionally and gets by without having to take three or four naps a day. Everyone says that T-cell ratios are such great markers for AIDS. Almost all our patients have T-cell increase on acupuncture and this seems to upset the physicians who follow them up elsewhere. One young doctor came up to see what we were doing and he got excited but when he came back, he reported that his director told him that T-cells were not that important and that exercise and nutrition were the major factor in the improvements we were getting. If the director really believes this, he should have a press conference and announce it so others can have the advantages of the same thing. Likewise, some hospitals keep asking us four or five times to give them our data but nothing ever comes from it. The idea that someone out of the medical mainstream might be helping these patients is upsetting to the physicians at the conventional centers.

Eighty percent of the time, patients who complain of weight loss, night sweats and lymphomatous type of symptoms start to improve by three treatments and acupuncture protects them against recurrent infections. A Lancet article a year or so ago mentions this. We have a patient with Cryptosporidiosis (which all the authorities say cannot be satisfactorily treated) but he did well and in four months he was clear, even by laboratory evidence. When I called up the city office to report on the case, the man I talked to dismissed it by saying that obviously the man did not have AIDS if he had responded . . . that he must have had sheep herder's disease . . . this in New York City!!

33

VITAMIN D—THE MISLABELED HORMONE

W ebster's dictionary defines a vitamin as "any of a number of unrelated complex organic substances found variously in most foods and essential in small amounts for the normal functioning of the body." There are indications that excessive milk drinking may be involved in arteriosclerosis and heart disease and that synthetic Vitamin D, with which all commercial milk is fortified, might also be implicated.

The discovery that codliver oil could prevent and cure rickets (a former scourge of infants and children in which their bones softened and deformed in wintertime and in areas of little sunlight) was one of the happy advances of medicine. It was eventually found that the active component of codliver oil is Calciferol (Vitamin D-3) which is also formed from cholesterol within the skin following exposure to sunlight.

An extensive review by Loomis in 1969 presented evidence that rickets is not a deficiency disease. Calciferol and ergasterol (a plant sterol known as Vitamin D-2, which, when irradiated with ultraviolet light has equal properties to the former) cannot be vitamins as previously assumed because: (1) Rickets cannot be induced in laboratory animals by feeding them a diet deficient in Vitamin D. It can only be produced by a diet with an unbalanced calcium and phosphorus ratio. (2) Rickets can be successfully treated in children by exposure to sunlight alone and Wurtman has shown that sunlight strongly and measurably enhances calcium uptake and utilization in adults in the winter time. It can be concluded that sunlight is not a vitamin nor are calciferol and ergosterol. The latter are growth promoting hormones essential to the proper metabolism of calcium within the body. They facilitate absorption of calcium from the intestines and interact with its metabolism within kidney, bone and muscle tissues.

The widespread use of Vitamin D, and especially the synthetic D-2 form, used in most vitamin mixtures and in the fortification of milk, may cause many illnesses of disturbed calcium and cholesterol metabolism and of conditions related to magnesium deficits. There have been pediatric reports of serious renal disease and disabilities connected with an elevated blood calcium; these include mental deficits, convulsions from magnesium deficiency, and increased susceptibility to environmental poisoning from lead and cadmium. Following the introduction of irradiated ergasterol in 1928, there has been an increasing incidence of pediatric disease tied to doses only slightly higher than the recommended daily dosage. In adults small excesses of ergasterol have been implicated in the formation of cataracts, arteriosclerosis, kidney stones and osteoporosis. Recently it has been shown that doses only slightly higher than the recommended daily allowance might be implicated in myocardial infarction evolving from a magnesium deficiency induced within the heart muscle. This production of cardiac necrosis is consistent with the laboratory studies of Dr. Hans Selye and of Dr. Mildred Seeley. A relationship of magnesium metabolism to myocardial infarction has been shown by the improved survival rates obtained when magnesium is given immediately to victims of myocardial infarcts.

The British Medical Association in 1950, the Canadian

Bulletin on Nutrition in 1953 and the American Academy of Pediatrics in 1963 and in 1965, recommended against the fortification of food with Vitamin D. This presumably referred to milk, whose intake in children and adults alike is uncontrolled. It is considered that codliver oil, which contains the natural substance identical to calciferol formed within the skin, is probably less toxic than the irradiated ergasterol so widely used in commercial vitamins and milk.

It is hoped that the FDA which has allowed the commercial exploitation of children's vitamins and milk, will eventually address itself to this problem. Vitamin D-2 is undoubtedly efficacious but its safety should be precisely determined.

34

DR. MARIA DE SOUSA

The intellectually stimulating work of Dr. Maria de Sousa and her team at Sloan Kettering Institute from 1977 to 1984 demonstrated that the immune system, (and particularly its T-lymphocytes) are intimately involved with iron metabolism.

Dr. de Sousa's elegant demonstrations, aligning to previous research in the metabolism of iron, have shown that deficiencies and defects of the immune system affect the transport, storage and utilization of iron within the body. Conversely, the presence of free iron in the body can, by its effects on lymphocytes, affect many disease states. The inter-relationships of the immune system and iron metabolism that are present in leukemia, Hodgkin's disease, malignancy and many infectious processes, suggest their involvement in the evolution of much degenerative disease.

Dr. de Sousa's work, suggesting that iron might interfere with optimal immunologic function and increase the growth of cancer cells, confirms previous work on the competition of microbes with body cells for iron; it may help explain the low serum iron levels often noted in AIDS patients who have no history of blood loss. What has long been viewed as women's pre-menopausal resistance to infection in comparison to men might be tied to their low iron content from monthly blood loss. There appears to be a narrow separation between the operating deficiencies of anemia and the reticuloendothelial depression of too much iron.

Dr. de Sousa's work is consistent with the conviction of many clinicians and nutritionists that the indiscriminate use of iron compounds in medicine, and the FDA-decreed inclusion of iron in all flour products, is probably a health hazard for many population groups. It suggests that, like Vitamin D-2, the compulsory inclusion of iron in our food supply is unsafe for certain segments of the population and possibly a factor in our increasing incidence of degenerative disease. It is an area that should be investigated, by either the FDA or Congress.

35

DR. MAX GERSON

Dr. Max Gerson was described by Dr. Albert Schweitzer (who, with his wife, was among Gerson's patients) as "the genius who walks among us". A refugee from Nazi Germany and the possessor of impeccable scientific credentials, Dr. Gerson applied diet to the healing of a wide range of degenerative disease, including tuberculosis and cancer. His thesis that a damaged liver is a primary precursor of degenerative disease is consistent with current concepts that liver status reflects the functional capacity of the reticuloendothelial system.

The basis of the Gerson regime is a comprehensive restoration of immunologic and metabolic function by a diet of organic vegetables, juiced and raw for the most part, the initial avoidance of meat in any form except for raw liver juice, and the elaborate and painstaking hourly program of a carefully prepared and administered diet. His detoxification of the body by coffee enemas has probably scandalized and perplexed orthodox practitioners more than any other item of his program, but has only affirmed this ancient naturopathic practice among the health-oriented. An academic study of the Gerson regime has reportedly concluded that it contains megadoses of minerals and vitamins.

Dr. Gerson was prominently mentioned in "Death Be Not Proud", John Gunther's moving tribute to his son, whose temporary remission of a brain tumor was achieved under Dr. Gerson's care. Because of Dr. Gerson's unorthodox approaches, he was expelled from the New York Medical Society, deprived of his hospital affiliations, and prominently included in the Cancer Society's "Unproven Methods of Cancer Management".

Modifications of the Gerson regime are found in almost all health oriented therapies, and a wider recognition of Dr. Gerson as one of the great physicians of his time appears likely. No one who dismisses his contributions has ever read his "A Cancer Therapy". Published in 1958, it outlines the fundamentals of almost every metabolic and nutritional concept used in Health Oriented Medicine.

EXCERPTS FROM "A CANCER THERAPY"*

"We must conclude that the soil and all that grows in it is not something distant from us but must be regarded as our external metabolism which produces the basic substances for our internal metabolism.

Cancer is a chronic degenerative disease where almost all essential organs are involved in the more advanced cases. . . .

The ideal task of cancer therapy is to restore the function of the oxidizing system . . . this involves: 1. detoxification of the whole body; 2. providing essential mineral contents of the potassium group; 3. adding oxidizing enzymes continuously. This will create a near normal condition of the oxidizing system to which malignant cells with the fermentation system cannot adapt.

The natural task of cancer therapy is to bring the body back to normal physiology or as near to it as is possible. The next task is to keep the physiology of the metabolism in that natural equilibrium. . . . I believe the surest way to achieve this is to restore to the body its ability to produce non-bacterial inflammatory reactions." (This last statement can apply equally well to AIDS today.).

---

*published by The Gerson Institute Box 430, Bonita CA. 92002

36

MACROBIOTICS

Within the past decade, the public has changed its former perception of Macrobiotics as a cult of brown rice health-nuts. It is now generally viewed as a nutritional discipline (primarily but not exclusively vegetarian) that can be pertinent and beneficial in many areas of health and illness.

Macrobiotics is a synthesis of Oriental philosophy, seeking primarily through diet to achieve a balanced integration of our internal and external environments. It is primarily concerned with balances (Yin-Yang, anabolic-catabolic, acid-alkaline, etc.). With broad philosophic parameters, the movement has cult overtones but it works for many and provides an orientation for others. Its philosophy and nutritional content, applicable to many chronic and degenerative conditions, appear beneficial for some AIDS patients, especially those in whom underlying damage has not been extensive. For these, Macrobiotics provides a background of detoxification and balance that may maintain the patients status quo or even enable the body to begin the healing process.

Macrobiotics has been credited with stabilizing Kaposi's sarcoma but total lesion regression attributable to diet alone is questionable. Many AIDS patients combine a macrobiotic routine with other therapeutic modalities, thus rendering any evaluation of individual components difficult. (If you are cut by a saw, which tooth did it?)

Strict adherence to macrobiotic precepts is neither simple nor easy. Macrobiotic cooking is time consuming and the ingredients for broad palatability are not always readily available. Maintaining a macrobiotic program requires stability, dedication and patience, so improvement rather than optimal results is most often achieved.

37

STAPHAGE LYSATE

In the late 1940s, Dr. Robert E. Lincoln noted that Staphage Lysate (SPL), a bacterial vaccine made from Staphylococci, when inhaled so that it was absorbed throughout the respiratory tract, was not only beneficial in sinus infection but improved or even cured a wide spectrum of illness. Ebuillient and resourceful, Dr. Lincoln developed a remarkable medical practice based largely on SPL. Wide public interest in the therapy and the rather far out theory that Dr. Lincoln propounded for its efficacy, so disturbed the Massachusetts Medical Society that it revoked his membership in that august organization.

Dr. Lincoln achieved national attention from a Congressional committee investigation of his therapy but the death of Senator Tobey at this time removed one of his most fervid supporters and Lincoln himself died of a heart attack two years later.

Since then, Staphage Lysate has been quietly manufactured and sold as a specific therapy for acute and chronic Staphylococcal infections. Unofficially, it has been widely used by pragmatic physicians who have had encouraging results in conditions as far ranging as allergies, arthritis, asthma, croup, Crohn's disease, multiple sclerosis, Herpes, warts and cancer. It is relatively inexpensive, almost totally non-toxic, and can be administered by inhalation, orally, and by injection.

A scientific rationale for the efficacy of SPL was unavailable in Dr. Lincoln's time but it is now accepted as a potent reticuloendothelial stimulant, especially of the T-lymphocytes. It also helps to induce the formation of Interferon and Interleukin I. The latter is the predecessor of Interleukin II, now prominently investigated in the therapy of AIDS and cancer. SPL can also be used as a skin test for cell-mediated immunity; the majority of adults, having had Staphylococcal infections, have a positive reaction.

SPL was long listed as unproven by the American Cancer Society, so it has had little serious investigation in the United States. Only its widespread and frequently surreptitious use has enabled it to survive as a practical, versatile and safe non-specific immunostimulant.

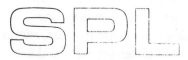

Delmont Laboratories, Inc.

UPDATE

Staphage Lysate (U.S. License 299)

Box AA / Swarthmore, PA 19081
(215) 543-3365

BIBLIOGRAPHY

General

Mudd S. JAMA 218(11): 1671-1673 (1971).
SPL elicits cell-mediated immunity.

Mudd S, Shayegani M. Ann NY Acad Sci 236: 244-251 (1974).

Clinical Research (Human)

Baker AG. Am Pract Dig Treat 9(4): 591-598 (1958).
SPL provides sustained symptomatic relief in chronic
bronchial asthma with no adverse reactions.

Baker AG. Pa Med J 66(Apr): 25-28 (1963).
SPL is a therapy of value and safety in treating staphylococcal diseases and complications in eight allergic patients.

..ss DW, et al. Ann Plastic Surg 6(5): 393-395 (1981).
SPL is a useful adjunct in the treatment of hidradenitis
suppurativa.

Mills AE. Laryngoscore 72(3): 367-383 (1962).
SPL is effective in preventing and controlling various
staphylococcal infections. Nonspecifically, SPL increases
the resistance to Gram-negative infection. (A 10-year study)*

Minami K, Ageo I. Clin Dermatol (Japan) 20(4): 249-254 (1978).
(English summary available)
SPL provides improvement in treating both flat warts and
ordinary warts.

Mudd S. JAMA 225(1): 65 (1973).
SPL provides specific cell-mediated immunity against
S. aureus, as well as nonspecific cell-mediated immunity
against a wide variety of intracellular pathogens in
staphylococcal-hypersensitized animals.

Mudd S; Baker AG. In Hasagawa T, ed. Proceedings of the First
Intersectional Congress of IAMS, vol 4, Science Council of Japan,
1975, pp 459-470.
SPL's elicitation of nonspecific cell-mediated immunity as
both a rational and promising therapy for herpesvirus and
aphthous ulcers.

Mudd S, Taubler JH, Baker AG. J Reticuloendothel Soc 8(5):
493-498 (1970).
The concept of induction-elicitation and its potential
clinical value.

Niimura M. Inoue Y, Kawashima M. Nishinihon J Dermatol (Japan)
42: in press (1980). (English summary available)
SPL is effective in treating adolescent flat warts.

Salmon GG Jr, Symonds M. J Med Soc NJ 60(May): 188-193 (1963).
SPL affords exceptionally good results in controlling
staphylococcal infections in 80% of 607 patients with no
significant adverse effects.

Tsuda S, et al. Nishinihon J Dermatol (Japan) 39(6): 942-948
(1977). (English tabular summary available)
SPL is effective in treating flat warts and ordinary warts.

Urabe H, et al. Nishinihon J Dermatol (Japan) 42(12): 289-296
(1980). (English translation available)
SPL is effective in treating virus-caused warts.

Vymola F, et al. Ann NY Acad Sci 236: 508-514 (1974).
SPL is effective in the treatment of staphylococcal
osteomyelitis.

Clinical Research (Veterinary)

Allbritton AR. Proc 1st Symp Vet Pharmacol Therap: 182-226 (1978).
SPL is effective in the treatment of a variety of derma-
tologic infections with staphylococcal involvement including
deep pyodermas.

Anderson RK. Comp CE Pract Vet 2(5): 361-371 (1980).
SPL is effective in the treatment of recurrent staphylococcal infections and/or hypersensitivity.

Pilarczyk JP. Canine Practice 8(1): 38-40 (1981).
SPL is an adjunct in the treatment of bacterial hypersensitivity.

Laboratory Research

Allen EG, Mudd S. Infec Immun 7(1): 62-67 (1973).
SPL provides resistance to vaccinia virus challenge in
staphylococcal-hypersensitized mice.

Dean JH, et al. J Immunol 115(4): 1060-1064 (1975).
SPL stimulates lymphoproliferation (B- and T-cells).

Esber HJ, Bogdon AE. Research by BD&G Mason Research Institute,
Worcester, MA 01608, 1978.
SPL as an adjunct to surgery effectively increased the number
of "cures" over surgery alone in a breast tumor model in
staphylococcal-hypersensitized rats.

Esber HJ, Bogdon AE. Research by BD&G Mason Research Institute,
Worcester, MA 01608, 1978.
SPL provides antitumor protection against Erlich's ascites
in staphylococcal-hypersensitized mice.

Esber HJ, De Courcy SJ Jr, Bogdon AE. J Immunopharmacol 3(1):
79-92 (1981).
SPL produces enhanced resistance to K. pneumoniae (30%
survival) and S. aureus (80-100% survival) infection in
staphylococcal-hypersensitized mice. SPL showed no anti-
tumor activity in mice implanted with Sarcoma-180 but
caused significant prolongation of survival with Erlich's
ascites.

Fujizoki Pharmaceutical Co., Ltd., Tokyo, Japan, 1980.
SPL shows no adverse pharmacologic effects.

Hirayama H, et al. Pharmacometrics (Japan) 20(3): 455-471
(1980). (English abstract available)
SPL causes no acute or subacute toxicity in rabbits.

-more-

38

ULTRAVIOLET IRRADIATION OF BLOOD

U ltraviolet irradiation of blood for conditions unresponsive to conventional treatment is another fascinating and neglected medical therapy. It was used for viral infections (Hepatitis, Polio, Mumps, Measles, and Herpes), bacterial infections poorly treated conventionally, inflammatory processes (nephritis, iritis, pancreatitis, thrombophlebitis, and arthritis), peripheral circulatory processes and other miscellaneous ailments.

The story began in the 1920s when Dr. E. Knott, a physiologist, followed up extensive European reseach into the systemic effects of ultraviolet skin irradiation. A number of investigators had felt that such effects might be mediated by blood concomittantly irradiated in the capillaries and veins within and below the skin. Knott and his colleague Edbloom, developed an instrument, within whose treatment chamber blood from heavily infected animals could be exposed to carefully monitored ultraviolet irradiation. The blood, reinjected into the animal from which it had been drawn, rendered the animal free of infection, even though it was unnecessary to expose the blood sufficiently to render it immediately sterile. They also found it was necessary to irradiate and re-inject only a small part of the animal's total blood volume to achieve beneficial results. It was presumed that the irradiated white blood cells instigated a chain reaction that stimulated the enzyme systems of the body. Especially evident was a marked increase in the oxygen carrying capacity of the blood, a general body detoxification (presumably from liver stimulation) and a modulation of the autonomic nervous system.

In the 1930s, the technique was used as desperation therapy for patients dying of overwhelming infections. The dramatic success of these cases led to a wide medical interest in the technique and over a hundred Knott blood irradiators were manufactured and distributed to physicians throughout the country.

For approximately twenty five years, observations and results from several thousand patients were summarized and presented at medical meetings and in major medical journals; blood irradiation as a part of medical practice gradually died out when antibiotics and other products of modern technology appeared. Despite the formation of the Foundation for Blood Irradiation, established by patients whose lives had been saved by the process and by the physicians who had used it, irradiation of blood completely faded from the medical scene by the 1970s. At this time, the FDA was given the power to control all medical equipment and devices, so the possibility of a revival of blood irradiation in this country dissolved.

Now, blood irradiation has resurfaced as a respectable medical therapy in Europe. The Germans have perfected a small and more efficient version of the Knott equipment and have organized a professional group called the INTERNATIONALE ARTZLICHE ARBEITGEMEINSCHAFT FUR HEMATO-GENE OXYDATIONSTHERAPIE. This abbreviates to IAA-HOT and the equipment is known as HOT equipment. The original Knott specifications for its use have been expanded so that ultraviolet blood irradiation covers the entire field of reticuloendothelial system stimulation, including the properdin system of protection against opportunistic infections. The ultraviolet rays also react with the oxygen used to push the blood through the equipment, and produce ozone, thus serving as an additional oxygenating factor in treating many conditions.

Again, the FDA's proof of efficacy requirements block from availability and use a treatment that is pertinent to many of our most serious health problems, including Herpes, Hepatitis, and AIDS.

FOUNDATION FOR BLOOD IRRADIATION, INC. —)efunct as of, the 70's

1 UBI Therapy is intravenously applied ultra-violet energy.

2 This produces in human beings effects of a profound basic nature, photochemical in some aspects, biochemical & physiological in many others.

3 These effects have proved to be clinically of great value in a wide variety of disease processes.

4 No harmful effects have been observed over a period of more than 25 years, during which UBI has been given more than 500,-000 times to over 30,000 patients by at least 100 physicians.

1 A rapid detoxifying effect, subsidence of toxic symptoms

2 An increase in venous oxygen, in patients with depressed blood oxygen values

3 A marked anti-inflammatory effect in diseases where severe damaging inflammatory processes exist

4 A powerful regulatory or normalizing effect on the autonomic nervous system, e.g. increased arteriolar flow is needed; relief of bronchospasm, paralytic ileus, pain of thrombophlebitis

5 A rapid rise in resistance to viral and bacterial infection, acute or chronic

CLINICAL EFFECTS OF UBI

EXCELLENT IN:

A Viral infections
1 Hepatitis: serum, infectious, acute, chronic
2 Atypical pneumonia
3 Acute poliomyelitis, encephalitis, myelitis
4 Mumps, measles, mononucleosis, herpes

B Bacterial infections
1 Septicemias: staphylococcus, streptococcus, pneumococcus, B. coli, salmonella
2 Pneumonias
3 Wound infections, lymphangitis, lymphadenitis
4 Peritonitis
5 Typhoid fever
6 Recurrent furunculosis, carbunculosis

C Profound overwhelming toxemias due to many fulminating disease processes (a life saving measure)

D Severe damaging inflammatory processes, e.g. *acute: thrombophlebitis, fibrositis, bursitis, nephritis, iritis, uveitis, cholecystitis, pancreatitis*

E Diseases due to inadequate peripheral circulation, e.g. *varicose and diabetic ulcer, peripheral atherosclerosis, some types of gangrene, vascular headache*

F Non-healing wounds, delayed union of fractures

G Subacute nephritis, early nephrosis

H Rheumatoid arthritis, with some patients obviously UBI sensitive, responding dramatically to UBI, others refractory to it; 70-75% aided by UBI

GOOD IN:

A Pemphigus

B Bronchiectasis, emphysema *(palliative effect in some patients)*

PARTIAL
BIBLIOGRAPHY

"Irradiated Blood Transfusion in The Treatment of Infections". *Northwest Med.*, 33:300. By V. K. Hancock and E. K. Knott, 1934.

"Ultraviolet Irradiation of Auto-Transfused Human Blood Studies in Oxygen Absorption Values". *Am. J. Med. Scs.* 197: No. 6,873, by George Miley, June 1939.

"Irradiation of Auto-Transfused Blood Ultraviolet Spectral Energy in 110 Cases". *M. Clin. North Am.* 24:723, by Henry A. Barrett, 1940.

"Method of Irradiating Circulating Blood in Vitro With Ultraviolet Spectral Energy; Studies of Its Physiological Effects in Vivo Applications in Humans". *Proceeding Am. Phys. Soc.*, by George P. Miley, April 1941.

"Ultraviolet Irradiation of Auto-Transfused" Blood in the Treatment of Puerperal Sepsis". *Am. J. Surg.*, 54: No. 3, 591, by E. W. Rebbeck, 1941.

"Knott Technic of Ultraviolet Blood Irradiation in Acute Pyogenic Infections". *N.Y.S. Jrl. Med.*, 42: No. 1, by Geo. Miley Jan. 1942.

"Ultraviolet Irradiation of Auto-Transfused Blood in the Treatment of Postabortional Sepsis." *Am. J. Surg.*, 55: No. 3, 46, by E. W. Rebbeck, March 1942.

"Syndrome of the Posterior Inferior Cerebellar Artery. *Arch. Otolarynge,*by A. Cinelli, July 1942.

"Treatment of Blood Stream Infections with Hemo-Irradiation". *Am. Jrl. Surg.*, 58 No. 3,336, by Virgil K. Hancock, Dec. 1942.

"Ultraviolet Blood Irradiation Therapy". *Transactions of Am. Therapy Soc.* Vol. 42 by George Miley, 1942.

"Double Septicemia Following Prostatectomy Treated by the Knott Technic of Ultra-Violet Blood Irradiation". *Am. J. of Surg.*, 57:536, by E. W. Rebbeck & R. A. Walther, 1942.

"Knott Technic of Ultraviolet Blood Irradiation as a Control of Infection in Peritonitis". *Rev. Gastroenterol*, 10: No. 1, 1-26, by Geo. P. Miley & Elmer W. Rebbeck, Jan.-Feb. 1943.

"Treatment of 8 Cases of Atypical Pneumonia by Ultraviolet Blood Irradiation". *Am. Bact. Soc.*, Penn. Chapter, by Geo. Miley, Feb. 1943.

"Ultraviolet Irradiation of Blood in the Treatment of Escherichia Coli Septicemia". *Arch. Therapy*, 24:158, by E. W. Rebbeck, March 1943.

"Preoperative Hemo-Irradiations". *Am. J. Surg.*, 61: No. 2, 259, by E. W. Rebbeck, 1943.

"Five Years Experience with Hemo-Irradiations". *Am. J. Surg.* 61:42, by Henry A. Barrett, 1943.

"Control of Acute Thrombophlebitis with Ultraviolet Blood Irradiation Therapy". *Am. J. Surg.*, 64:313, by George Miley, 1943.

"Present Status of Ultraviolet Blood Irradiation (Knott Technic)". *Arch. of Phys. Therapy*, 25:375, by Geo. P. Miley, June 1944.

"Efficacy of Ultraviolet Blood Irradiation Therapy in the Control of Staphylococcemias". *Am. J. Surg.*, 64: No. 3,313, by George P. Miley, June 1944.

"Ultraviolet Blood Irradiation Therapy (Knott Technic) in Non-Healing Wounds". *Am. J. Surg.*, 65: No. 3, 368, by Geo. P. Miley, Sept. 1944.

"Ultraviolet Irradiation Relative to Anoxia and Bends Susceptibility". *U.S. Nav. M. Bul.*, 43:37-X, by William M. Davidson 1944.

"Ultraviolet Blood Irradiation Therapy in Acute Poliomyelitis". *Archives of Phys. Therapy*, 25:651, by Geo. P. Miley, Nov. 1944.

"Ultraviolet Blood Irradiation Therapy of Apparently Intractable Bronchial Asthma". *Arch. Phys.*, 27:24, by G. P. Miley, R. E. Seidel, J. A. Christensen, Jan. 1946.

"Recovery From Botulism Coma Following Ultraviolet Blood Irradiation (Knott Technic)". *Rev. Gastroentrol*, 13: No. 1, 17, by Geo. P. Miley, Jan.-Feb. 1946.

"The Effect of Short Time Ultraviolet Irradiation on Blood and Biochemical Compounds". by Morton Beroza, May 1946.

"Ultraviolet Blood Irradiation in Biliary Disease (Knott Method)". *Am. J. Surg.*, 70: No. 2. 235, by R. C. Olney, Aug. 1946.

"Ultraviolet Blood Irradiation Therapy in Acute Virus and Virus-Like Infections". *Rev. Gastroenterol*, 15: No. 4, 271, by Geo. P. Miley & J. Christensen, Apr. 1948.

"Development of Ultraviolet Blood Irradiation," *Am. Jrl. Surg.*, Vol. 76, No. 2, Aug. 1948, by E. K. Knott, D. Sc.

"Ultraviolet Blood Irradiation Therapy (Knott Technic) in Thrombophlebitis". *Am. J. Surg.*, 78: No. 6, 892, by G. P. Miley and P. M. Dunning, 1949.

"Uses of Ultraviolet Blood Irradiation Therapy (Knott Technic) in Atypical or Virus Type Pneumonia". By H. T. Lewis, Jr., June 1949.

"Use of Ultraviolet Blood Irradiation in Typhoid Fever". *Rev. of Gastroentrol*, 16: No. 8, 640, by E. W. Rebbeck & H. T. Lewis Jr., Aug. 1949.

"Ultraviolet Blood Irradiation in the Treatment of Acute Poliomyelitis". *Am. Blood Irradiation Soc., Bul.* 3: No. 3, by Frederick Burke, Albert A. Laverne, G. J. P. Barger, May 15, 1950.

"Treatment of Acute and Chronic X-ray Burns with Ultraviolet Blood Irradiation (Knott Technic)". By V. Hancock, June 1950.

"Use of Ultraviolet Blood Irradiation (Knott Technic in Biliary Tract Surgery". *Am. J. Surg.*, 80: No. 1, 108, by E. W. Rebbeck, July 1950.

"Ultraviolet Blood Irradiation Therapy (Knott Technic) in Rheumatic Fever in Children". *Exp. and Surg.*, 8: No. 1, by V. P. Wasson, G. P. Miley & P. M. Dunning, 1950.

"Use of Ultraviolet Blood Irradiation in the Treatment of Bursitis & Tendinitis Calcarea". *Am. J. Surg.*, 81: No. 6, 622, by Floyd Neff & C. M. Anderson, June 1951.

"Uvetis". *Jackson Clinic Bul.*, 13: No. 4, by Albert L. Rhoades, 1951.

"Observation — June 1951". By Lowell A. Erf, Jefferson Med. Col. Phil. Pa.

"Use of Hemo-Irradiation (Knott Technique) in eye infections". *Ind. and Surg.*, 21:4, by Donald Farmer, Clifford P. Sullivan, William B. Sullivan, April 1952.

"Preventing Amputation from Diabetic Gangrene". By R. C. Olney, June 1952.

"Effectiveness of Ultraviolet Blood Irradiation Therapy in Virus and Virus-like Diseases", *Newsletter, Am. Blood Irradiation Soc.* Feb. 1953, Bul., 6: No. 1.

"Control of Deltoid Bursitis with the Knott Technic of Blood Irradiation Therapy". *Am. J. Surg.*, 86: No. 4, 401, by G. P. Miley & A. A. Laplume, Oct. 1953.

"Treatment of Viral Hepatitis with the Knott Technic of Blood Irradiation". *Am. J. Surg.*, 90, No. 3, 402, by R. C. Olney, Sept. 1955.

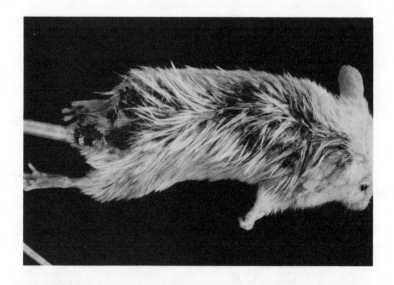

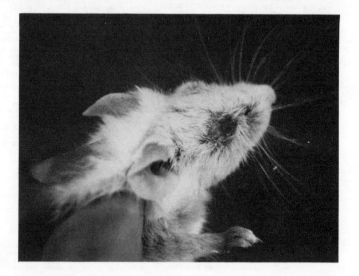

Wirostko and Johnson's mice injected with uveal fluid from collagen disease patients.

EPILOGUE

The AIDS problem is not confined only to medical research, nor will it necessarily be solved by allocating more money to expand an already enormous accumulation of unsorted and unused medical knowledge. The problem is not limited to the means of confining AIDS to those groups now recognized as at greatest risk nor is it the resolution of the current bewilderment and confusion of the general public. The latter's general inhumanity against those whose lives have been touched by the disease stems from ignorance and is capable of a slow resolution as the medical picture clears.

The treatment of those with AIDS will be facilitated by medical recognition that AIDS is not the sole result of an infection with the AIDS virus but is a constellation of signs and symptoms of a body specifically deranged by severe stresses. These include viruses, bacteria, fungi and parasites, with the AIDS virus as the precipitating organism. Recognition that it is a systemic disease of multiple causes will restore attention to the medical treatment of the whole patient and not just the T-lymphocytes dysfunction or whatever infection presents.

Public frustrations and fears from the many words but few beneficial results in AIDS parallel their apprehension at the increase of cancer and its generally inadequate treatment. Pressure from the public at the political level may lead to a balanced appraisal and action by Congress in revising the FDA'S "proof of efficacy" requirements, the single greatest weight on American medicine today. Imposed by well meant legislation of the 1960s, it has been a mistake that has eliminated or blocked from the market many products that are urgently needed by American medicine.

This action at the political level would help reconcile many areas of conventional and alternative medical practices. It would correct the presumption that health and medical practices, even when based on authority, can be legislatively guaranteed effective. Pressure from all segments of a concerned public can also encourage and expand the horizons of even the most specialized researchers and clinicians in AIDS, cancer and degenerative disease. This will include a more open approach to pertinent areas of uninvestigated medical research, especially that represented by pleomorphic organisms and the Naessens microscope. Last, but not least, there will be a realization that the physical components of medical science are insufficient by themselves.

Scientific medicine, the fusion of the physical sciences and 20th century technology must reestablish a working alignment with the biologic aspects of Health Oriented Medicine from which it evolved. The current AIDS impasse displays that the capabilities of both are optimum when they work together and are allied to the ancient concepts of Holistic Medicine, emphasizing mind, spirit, and biologic energies. The volume of health and medical knowledge available from all three areas is now so vast that it can be neither encompassed nor controlled by any one discipline.

The Trizoid and not the three separate and overlapping spheres referred to in Chapter III, is the form of the emerging medical future. It is a circle, twisted upon itself and folded to form three ovoid leaves whose individual integrity is bound to a shared center. Their relationships are such that none can stand alone, and the violation of even an unshared border destroys the integrity of the entire circle from which each segment is formed and defined. The Trizoid resolves the competition of the overlapping but separate spheres of medicine; Scientific, Health Oriented and Holistic Medicine are immutably joined, each are insufficient by themselves but are essential to complete the other's potentials. The most effective approach to the prevention and the treatment of AIDS, cancer, and other degenerative diseases will be found allied within the Trizoid concept.

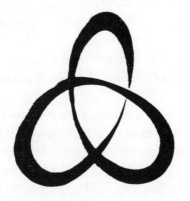

INDEX